Committee on Military Nutrition Research

Activity Report

**December 1, 1994
through
May 31, 1999**

AF172861

Food and Nutrition Board
INSTITUTE OF MEDICINE

Prepared by

Mary I. Poos, Rebecca Costello, and Sydne J. Carlson-Newberry

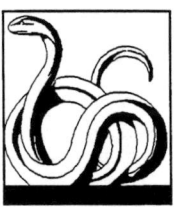

NATIONAL ACADEMY PRESS
Washington, D.C. 1999

NATIONAL ACADEMY PRESS • 2101 Constitution Avenue, N.W. • Washington, DC 20418

NOTICE: The project that is the subject of this report was approved by the Governing Board of the National Research Council, whose members are drawn from the councils of the National Academy of Sciences, the National Academy of Engineering, and the Institute of Medicine. The members of the committee responsible for the report were chosen for their special competences and with regard for appropriate balance.

The Institute of Medicine was established in 1970 by the National Academy of Sciences to enlist distinguished members of the appropriate professions in the examination of policy matters pertaining to the health of the public. In this, the Institute acts under both the Academy's 1863 congressional charter responsibility to be an adviser to the federal government and its own initiative in identifying issues of medical care, research, and education. Dr. Kenneth I. Shine is president of the Institute of Medicine.

This report presents a summary of activities of the Committee on Military Nutrition Research (CMNR) and its Subcommittee on Body Composition, Nutrition, and Health of Military Women (BCNH) from December 1, 1994, through May 31, 1999. All of the activities mentioned here have resulted in reports that were previously published or submitted as letter reports to the sponsor and as such were reviewed by a group other than the authors according to procedures approved by a Report Review Committee consisting of members of the National Academy of Sciences, the National Academy of Engineering, and the Institute of Medicine. This activities summary has not been separately reviewed and represents an overview of all activities during the project period as designated.

The activities of the Committee on Military Nutrition Research (CMNR) from December 1, 1994, through May 31, 1999, were supported by grant DAMD17-94-J-4046 from the U.S. Army Medical Research and Materiel Command. The activities of the Subcommittee on Body Composition, Nutrition, and Health of Military Women (BCNH) from August 15, 1995 to September 30, 1998, were supported by grant DAMD17-95-1-5037 from the U.S. Army Medical Research and Materiel Command. A separate report on the activities of the BCNH Subcommittee was submitted in June 1998.

This report is available for sale from:

National Academy Press
2101 Constitution Avenue, N.W.
Lock Box 285
Washington, DC 20055

Call (800) 626-6242 or (202) 334-3313 (in the Washington metropolitan area), or visit the NAP's on-line bookstore at *www.nap.edu.*

For more information about the Institute of Medicine and the Food and Nutrition Board, visit the IOM's and FNB's home pages at *www.national-academies.org/iom* and *www.national-academies.org/iom/fnb.*

Copyright 1999 by the National Academy of Sciences. All rights reserved.

Printed in the United States of America.

The serpent has been a symbol of long life, healing, and knowledge among almost all cultures and religions since the beginning of recorded history. The image adopted as a logotype by the Institute of Medicine is based on a relief carving from ancient Greece, now held by the Staatliche Museen in Berlin.

COMMITTEE ON MILITARY NUTRITION RESEARCH
(in December 1994)

ROBERT O. NESHEIM (*Chair*), Salinas, California

RICHARD L. ATKINSON, Departments of Medicine and Nutritional Sciences, University of Wisconsin, Madison

WILLIAM R. BEISEL, Department of Immunology and Infectious Diseases, The Johns Hopkins University School of Hygiene and Public Health, Baltimore, Maryland

GAIL E. BUTTERFIELD, Division of Endocrinology, Gerontology, and Metabolism, Stanford University School of Medicine and Geriatric Research, Education, and Clinical Center, Veterans Affairs Medical Center, Palo Alto, California

JOHN D. FERNSTROM, Department of Psychiatry, Pharmacology, and Neuroscience, University of Pittsburgh School of Medicine, Pennsylvania

JOËL A. GRINKER, Program in Human Nutrition, School of Public Health, University of Michigan, Ann Arbor

G. RICHARD JANSEN, Department of Food Science and Human Nutrition, Colorado State University, Fort Collins

ORVILLE A. LEVANDER, Vitamin and Mineral Nutrition Laboratory, U.S. Department of Agriculture Beltsville Human Nutrition Research Center, Beltsville, Maryland

GILBERT A. LEVEILLE, Nabisco Brands Incorporated, East Hanover, New Jersey

JOHN E. VANDERVEEN, Office of Plant and Dairy Foods and Beverages, Food and Drug Administration, Washington, D.C.

Food and Nutrition Board Liaison

JOHANNA T. DWYER, Frances Stern Nutrition Center and Department of Medicine, Tufts University and New England Medical Center Hospital, Boston, Massachusetts

U.S. Army Grant Officer Representative

JAMES A. VOGEL, U.S. Army Research Institute of Environmental Medicine, Natick, Massachusetts

Staff

BERNADETTE M. MARRIOTT, Program Director

DONNA F. ALLEN, Project Assistant

SUSAN M. KNASIAK, Project Assistant

iii

COMMITTEE ON MILITARY NUTRITION RESEARCH
(Current)

JOHN E. VANDERVEEN (*Chair*), Rockville, Maryland

LAWRENCE E. ARMSTRONG, Departments of Physiology and Neurobiology, and Exercise Science, University of Connecticut, Storrs

GAIL E. BUTTERFIELD, Nutrition Studies, Palo Alto Veterans Affairs Health Care System and Program in Human Biology, Stanford University, Palo Alto, California

WANDA L. CHENOWETH, Department of Food Science and Human Nutrition, Michigan State University, East Lansing

JOHN D. FERNSTROM, Department of Psychiatry, Pharmacology, and Neuroscience, University of Pittsburgh School of Medicine, Pennsylvania

ROBIN B. KANAREK, Department of Psychology, Tufts University, Boston, Massachusetts

ORVILLE A. LEVANDER, Nutrient Requirements and Functions Laboratory, U.S. Department of Agriculture Beltsville Human Nutrition Research Center, Beltsville, Maryland

ESTHER M. STERNBERG, Chief, Neuroendocrine Immunology and Behavior Section, National Institute of Mental Health, Bethesda, Maryland

Food and Nutrition Board Liaison

JOHANNA T. DWYER, Frances Stern Nutrition Center, New England Medical Center Hospital and Departments of Medicine and Community Health, Tufts Medical School and School of Nutrition Science and Policy, Boston, Massachusetts

U.S. Army Grant Officer Representative

LTC KARL E. FRIEDL, Military Operational Medicine Program, U.S. Army Medical Research and Materiel Command, Fort Detrick, Frederick, Maryland

Staff

MARY I. POOS (*from May 23, 1998*), Study Director

MARIZA SILVA (*from August 31, 1998*), Senior Project Assistant

FOOD AND NUTRITION BOARD
(in December 1994)

JANET C. KING (*Chair*), Department of Nutritional Sciences, University of California, Berkeley

EDWIN L. BIERMAN (*Vice Chair*), Division of Metabolism, Endocrinology, and Nutrition, University of Washington School of Medicine, Seattle

JOHN W. ERDMAN, JR. (*Vice Chair*), Division of Nutritional Sciences, University of Illinois, Urbana

CUTBERTO GARZA (*Vice Chair*), Division of Nutritional Sciences, Cornell University, Ithaca, New York

PERRY L. ADKISSON, Department of Entomology, Texas A&M University, College Station

LINDSAY H. ALLEN, Department of Nutrition, University of California, Davis

DENNIS M. BIER, Children's Nutrition Research Center, Baylor College of Medicine, Houston, Texas

FERGUS M. CLYDESDALE, Department of Food Science and Nutrition, University of Massachusetts, Amherst

HECTOR F. DeLUCA, Department of Biochemistry, University of Wisconsin, Madison

MICHAEL P. DOYLE, Department of Food Science and Technology, University of Georgia, Athens

JOHANNA T. DWYER, Frances Stern Nutrition Center and Department of Medicine, Tufts University and New England Medical Center Hospital, Boston, Massachusetts

SCOTT M. GRUNDY, University of Texas Southwestern Medical Center, Dallas

K. MICHAEL HAMBIDGE, Center for Human Nutrition, University of Colorado Health Sciences Center, Denver

LAURENCE N. KOLONEL, Epidemiology Program, Cancer Center of Hawaii, University of Hawaii, Honolulu

SANFORD A. MILLER, Graduate School of Biomedical Sciences, University of Texas Health Science Center, San Antonio

ALFRED SOMMER, The Johns Hopkins University School of Hygiene and Public Health, Baltimore, Maryland

VERNON R. YOUNG, Laboratory of Human Nutrition, School of Science, Massachusetts Institute of Technology, Cambridge

STEVE L. TAYLOR (*Ex-Officio*), Department of Food Science and Technology, University of Nebraska, Lincoln

ARTHUR H. RUBENSTEIN (*IOM Council Liaison*), Department of Medicine, The University of Chicago, Illinois

Staff
ALLISON A. YATES, Director
BERNADETTE M. MARRIOTT, Associate Director
GAIL E. SPEARS, Administrative Assistant
JAMAINE L. TINKER, Financial Associate

FOOD AND NUTRITION BOARD
(Current)

CUTBERTO GARZA (*Chair*), Division of Nutrition, Cornell University, Ithaca, New York

JOHN W. ERDMAN, JR. (*Vice Chair*), Division of Nutritional Sciences, College of Agriculture, University of Illinois at Urbana-Champaign

LINDSAY H. ALLEN, Department of Nutrition, University of California, Davis

BENJAMIN CABALLERO, Center for Human Nutrition, The Johns Hopkins University School of Hygiene and Public Health, Baltimore, Maryland

FERGUS M. CLYDESDALE, Department of Food Science, University of Massachusetts, Amherst

ROBERT J. COUSINS, Center for Nutritional Sciences, University of Florida, Gainesville

JOHANNA T. DWYER, Frances Stern Nutrition Center, New England Medical Center Hospital and Departments of Medicine and Community Health, Tufts Medical School and School of Nutrition Science and Policy, Boston, Massachusetts

SCOTT M. GRUNDY, Center for Human Nutrition, University of Texas Southwestern Medical Center at Dallas

CHARLES H. HENNEKENS, Harvard Medical School and Division of Preventive Medicine, Brigham and Women's Hospital, Boston, Massachusetts

SANFORD A. MILLER, Graduate School of Biomedical Sciences, University of Texas Health Science Center, San Antonio

ROSS L. PRENTICE, Division of Public Health Sciences, Fred Hutchinson Cancer Research Center, Seattle, Washington

A. CATHARINE ROSS, Department of Nutrition, The Pennsylvania State University, University Park

ROBERT E. SMITH, R. E. Smith Consulting, Inc., Newport, Vermont

VIRGINIA A. STALLINGS, Division of Gastroenterology and Nutrition, The Children's Hospital of Philadelphia, Pennsylvania

VERNON R. YOUNG, Laboratory of Human Nutrition, School of Science, Massachusetts Institute of Technology, Cambridge

STEVE L. TAYLOR (*Ex-Officio*), Department of Food Science and Technology and Food Processing Center, University of Nebraska, Lincoln

Staff
ALLISON A. YATES, Director
GAIL E. SPEARS, Administrative Assistant
GARY WALKER, Financial Associate

vii

Preface

The issues addressed in this report as well as in the previous activity report, *Committee on Military Nutrition Research Activity Report April 1, 1992– November 30, 1994* (IOM, 1994a), illustrate the diversity of activities addressed by the Committee on Military Nutrition Research (CMNR, the committee). This diversity has required the use of a broad range of expertise to respond to the issues brought to the CMNR. The range of scientific disciplines represented on the CMNR has been augmented as necessary through the use of workshops or special advisors to enable the CMNR to bring the degree and breadth of expertise necessary to properly respond to the subject under review. The committee has been pleased with and is very appreciative of the willing participation of the invited participants in these sessions and of their provision of written papers, which have constituted a major part of the CMNR reports. Many of these workshops have included experts from within the military who have shared their research activities and information. They have been excellent representatives of the quality of research conducted by the military on many of these problems.

The military is to be commended for continuing to ensure that the nutritional needs of its personnel are adequately met during the stress of military operations through its support of nutrition and related research. There has also been interest and support for modifications of rations of military personnel consistent with the advice provided by the nutrition and public health leadership in the United States. The CMNR is cognizant of the desire to balance long-term health considerations with the demands of maintaining performance under the environmental extremes of military operations.

The ability of operational rations to help sustain military performance has been the subject of CMNR review since 1982. Field studies have shown nutrient intake, other than calories, is sufficient to maintain the weight and performance of troops in the field. Complex interactions involving palatability of the ration components, convenience, fluid intake, socialization, and physical and psychological stresses that influence the consumption of operational rations are discussed in the publication, *Not Eating Enough, Overcoming Underconsumption of Operational Rations* (IOM, 1995a). Further evaluation of these complex factors are reviewed in the reports, *Military Strategies for Sustainment of Nutrition and Immune Function in the Field* (IOM, 1999b), *The Role of Protein and Amino Acids in Sustaining and Enhancing Performance* (IOM, 1999c), and the letter report on *Antioxidants and Oxidative Stress in Military Personnel* (February 12, 1999) and will undoubtedly continue to be of interest to the military and the CMNR.

We appreciate the close working relationships with James A. Vogel, who is now retired; Harris R. Lieberman, who replaced him at the Military Nutrition Division (currently the Military Nutrition and Biochemistry Division) at the U.S. Army Research Institute of Environmental Medicine; and LTC Karl E. Friedl of the U.S. Army Medical Research and Materiel Command for the excellent liaison they have provided between the military and the committee. They greatly assisted the work of the committee by bringing issues forward for consideration and helping to identify expertise familiar with these problems, particularly from within the Armed Forces.

As chair, I express my deep appreciation to all of the committee members past (Richard L. Atkinson, William R. Beisel, Joël A. Grinker, G. Richard Jansen, Gilbert A. Leveille, Douglas W. Wilmore) and present who have given their time, dedication, and expertise to the careful analysis of the issues and to developing the conclusions and recommendations of the committee. I would especially like to thank Dr. Robert O. Nesheim, who retired as Chair of the committee in June 1998, for providing the strong and thoughtful leadership for CMNR since its inception in 1982. He is a hard act to follow. I also thank all participants in the many workshops who have greatly aided our activities and assured that the appropriate expertise has been available to the committee.

Finally, I wish to express my appreciation to the staff of the Food and Nutrition Board assigned to this activity over the past 5 years. In particular I acknowledge for myself and the entire committee the outstanding support presently provided to this activity by Mary I. Poos, study director and Mariza Silva, project assistant. I also extend my sincere appreciation to Rebecca B. Costello, former study director; Bernadette M. Marriott, former study director; Sydne J. Carlson-Newberry, former program officer; Susan M. Knasiak-Raley, former research assistant; Melissa L. Van Doren, former project assistant; and Donna F. Allen, former project assistant. They have worked with extreme dedication to update and complete publication of several pending CMNR reports and to assure a timely response to the issues currently under consideration by the committee.

John E. Vanderveen, Ph.D.
Chair

Contents

Summary

The activities of the Food and Nutrition Board's Committee on Military Nutrition Research (CMNR, the committee) have been supported since 1994 by grant DAMD17-94-J-4046 from the U.S. Army Medical Research and Materiel Command (USAMRMC). This report fulfills the final reporting requirement of the grant, and presents a summary of activities for the grant period from December 1, 1994 through May 31, 1999. During this grant period, the CMNR has met from three to six times each year in response to issues that are brought to the committee through the Military Nutrition and Biochemistry Division of the U.S. Army Research Institute of Environmental Medicine at Natick, Massachusetts, and the Military Operational Medicine Program of USAMRMC at Fort Detrick, Maryland. The CMNR has submitted five workshop reports (plus two preliminary reports), including one that is a joint project with the Subcommittee on Body Composition, Nutrition, and Health of Military Women; three letter reports, and one brief report, all with recommendations, to the Commander, U.S. Army Medical Research and Materiel Command, since September 1995 and has a brief report currently in preparation. These reports are summarized in the following activity report with synopses of additional topics for which reports were deferred pending completion of military research in progress. This activity report includes as appendixes the conclusions and recommendations from the nine reports and has been prepared in a fashion to allow rapid access to committee recommendations on the topics covered over the time period.

To present a complete synopsis of CMNR activities, this report also includes two reports prepared by the Subcommittee on Body Composition, Nutrition, and Health of Military Women under grant DAMD17-95-1-5037 from the U.S. Army Medical Research and Materiel Command.

1

Background and Introduction

HISTORY OF THE COMMITTEE

The Committee on Military Nutrition Research (CMNR, the committee) was established in October 1982 in response to a request from the Assistant Surgeon General of the U.S. Army. It was first organized within the Food and Nutrition Board (FNB) of the National Research Council's (NRC) Commission on Life Sciences and in 1988 moved with the FNB to its new administrative home in the Institute of Medicine.

The committee's mission is to advise the U.S. Department of Defense on the need for and conduct of nutrition research and related issues. Specifically, the committee's tasks are:

- to identify nutritional factors that may critically influence the physical and mental performance of military personnel under all environmental extremes,
- to identify deficiencies in the existing database,
- to recommend research that would remedy these deficiencies as well as approaches for studying the relationship of diet to physical and mental performance, and
- to review and advise on standards for military feeding systems.

Within this context, the CMNR was asked to focus on nutrient requirements for performance during operational missions and deployment rather than requirements for military personnel in garrison, because the latter were judged not to differ significantly from those of the civilian population.

Although the composition of the committee changes through a 3-year rotation policy, the disciplines represented have consistently included human nutrition, nutritional biochemistry, performance physiology, immunology, food science, and psychology.

3

A subcommittee of the CMNR was established to review existing military policies governing body composition and fitness as well as postpartum return-to-duty standards, Military Recommended Dietary Allowances, and physical activity and nutritional practices to determine their individual and collective impact on the health, fitness, and readiness of active-duty women under a Defense Women's Health Research Program grant. In addition to several members of the parent committee, individuals with expertise in body composition assessment, physical fitness and performance, pregnancy and lactation, women's nutrition, weight management, epidemiology and survey design, and cognitive performance were included. This subcommittee was designated the Subcommittee on Body Composition, Nutrition, and Health of Military Women (BCNH committee). In addition, a group of individuals representing the body composition, fitness, and nutrition research and policy making bodies of the Army, Navy, and Air Force were invited by the sponsor to form a liaison panel to advise the BCNH committee.

Although this subcommittee operated under a separate grant, the two reports they prepared: *Assessing Readiness in Military Women: The Relationship of Body Composition, Nutrition, and Health* and *Reducing Stress Fractures in Physically Active Military Women* are included in this activity report for completeness.

COMMITTEE PROCEDURES

Meetings

Meetings have been of three types. *Full committee meetings* are scheduled at the request of the Army to review nutrition programs, food products, and specific research projects in various stages of development. At these meetings, oral presentations by Army personnel are augmented by written background material on one or more specific items for the Committee on Military Nutrition Research to review. The CMNR subsequently meets in executive session to discuss the materials and write a report to the Army that includes a summary of findings and recommendations. These reports are in the form of letters with attached supporting materials or brief, bound reports. *Subcommittee meetings* are convened by the committee chair either to plan future work, write reports, or, at the request of the Army, provide on-site review of research projects where the expertise of the entire committee membership is not required. Reports drafted by subcommittees of the CMNR are subject to the review and approval of the entire committee membership prior to completion. *Workshop meetings* are planned when issues have been presented to the CMNR by the Army that require broader expertise than exists within the committee, or for which the committee would like additional information or opinions. A CMNR workshop includes presentations from Army and other experts in nutrition and related sciences on an issue relevant to military nutrition research. The invited speakers are chosen for their specific expertise in the topic areas of concern and are asked to provide in-depth reviews of their area of expertise as it directly applies to a series of questions drafted by the sponsor. Speakers subsequently submit written versions of their presentations. These workshops thus provide additional state-of-the-art scientific information for the committee to consider in their evaluation of the issues at hand. At the conclusion of the presentations, the committee meets in executive session to discuss the issues and prepare conclusions and recommendations to be included as part of a book-style workshop report for subsequent release to the sponsors and the public.

If a topic is presented by the military where the committee membership does not feel that they can adequately cover the scientific range required, special advisors may be invited to augment the committee expertise and interact with the membership for a specific report. If the committee chair sees that expertise continues to be needed in a specific scientific area, a new member with expertise in that scientific discipline may be added to the committee through the normal 3-year rotation process.

Document Format

In 1992, the CMNR formalized the document format types that they used for their reports and developed a standardized report cover. This standardized cover presents a "series effect" to the CMNR reports and makes them readily identifiable as committee projects. Currently, there are four document formats used by the CMNR that reflect the specific needs of the Army. In 1994, the CMNR created a style guide to be used in future reports. This style was so well received that others in IOM have incorporated some aspects of it into their reports.

1. *Letter with attachments.* This type of document is prepared in response to a specific request from the Army for a review of a research project or program that requires a rapid response to be effective. The document must be a short, specific statement of recommendations directed to the Army command for rapid action. These items are research projects that are in progress or specific nutritional concerns that have abruptly arisen. The CMNR is presented orally with the findings and provided with the limited documentation available. The timeliness as well as the concise, highly specific, and confidential nature of these documents is specified by the Army when the item is presented to the CMNR. Three examples of letter reports are included in this activity report.

2. *Brief report with documentation.* This document format is typically used in response to a request for review of a food product, packaging process, completed research project, or planned educational program. The Army

provides an oral presentation as well as extensive documentation or product specifications. The time frame for the committee deliberations is several months, and the summary and recommendations are bound to the specifications to provide a clear understanding of the iteration of the product, process, project, or program that was reviewed. The 1996 CMNR report, *Pennington Biomedical Research Center September 1996 Site Visit*, is an example of a brief report (see p. 25 and Appendix G) as is the 1999 report (in progress) on *Caffeine Formulations for Sustainment of Mental Performance*.

3. *Workshop proceedings with summary and recommendations.* The Army identifies for the committee at least one topic each year for which they require a thorough review of the current literature by experts in the scientific field coupled with the committee's recommendations. This requirement is met with a workshop at which experts are asked to make oral presentations that include an overview of the literature and address specific questions posed by the Army. CMNR staff compile literature reviews and organize these meetings in close collaboration with the sponsor. The CMNR reviews these presentations and writes a detailed summary and recommendations to the Army. The resulting document includes the committee's findings with the presentations. The expected turn-around time for this document type is within 12 to 24 months. Examples of workshop reports are the committee's most recently released books, *Military Strategies for Sustainment of Nutrition and Immune Function in the Field* (May, 1999; see p. 45 and Appendix L), and *The Role of Protein and Amino Acids in sustaining and Enhancing Performance* (June, 1999; see p. 49 and Appendix M).

4. *Periodic activities reports.* The CMNR is also expected to prepare a bound report at variable intervals (3–5 years) that is a summation of the activities undertaken. No new information is presented in these reports. Typically these reports reflect contract periods and serve as a final report for the contract or contract renewal. This report is an example of the periodic activity report of the CMNR.

Document Review

In accordance with NRC guidelines, each report (with the exception of the activity reports) is reviewed in confidence by a separate, scientific review group. In 1992 the CMNR established a separate Review Panel to facilitate the rapid review of committee reports. When a report is begun, the panel members are alerted and polled as to who among them would be available to review the report. Typically, each report is reviewed by five to seven panel members. Additionally, three to five supplemental reviewers with expertise in the specific area being covered in a report may be approached, as was the case with the report, *Emerging Technologies for Nutrition Research* (IOM, 1997). The Review Panel members all have some experience with military nutrition and health issues and therefore have a basic understanding of the concepts under consideration. None are military personnel or have contracts with the military. The Review Panel has facilitated the speed of report review because the participants are interested and knowledgeable about the issues that come before the committee. In addition, as panel members they are prepared to consider reviewing reports with a rapid turn-around time. As with all NRC report reviews, the comments of the Review Panel are anonymous.

The committee then reviews the anonymous comments of this Review Panel and incorporates their suggestions where appropriate. Staff then write a response to the reviewers comments with a revised report draft and obtain final approval of the report from the Review Coordinator. Each Committee on Military Nutrition Research report is thus a thoughtfully developed presentation that incorporates the scientific opinion of the CMNR and the comments of National Research Council external reviewers.

ORGANIZATION OF THIS REPORT

This summary of the activities of the Committee on Military Nutrition Research reflects the period of performance from December 1, 1994 through May 31, 1999 supported by grant DAMD17-94-J-4046 from the U.S. Army Medical Research and Materiel Command to the Food and Nutrition Board for the CMNR program. It also includes the activities of the Subcommittee on Body Composition, Nutrition and Health which functioned in this time period. This report has been organized in topical fashion because the committee was requested on occasion to participate in reviews of research projects or products during several stages of their development over the course of this grant period. Activities are presented in the same order they were submitted to the sponsor.

A full listing of all committee meetings and members during the grant period are included as Appendixes A and B. At a number of meetings, the CMNR was presented with oral and written reports of research projects in progress or products under development. In a number of instances, the committee deferred a full review of these items until the project was complete. Summaries are provided in the body of this report of all activities in which the committee was requested to participate from December 1, 1994 through May 31, 1999, regardless of whether a report with recommendations was developed. In the appendixes, full copies of each letter report are included in the order mentioned in the text. For the brief reports and workshop reports, due to length, only the committee conclusions and recommendations have been included in the appendixes.

Not Eating Enough: Overcoming Underconsumption of Military Operational Rations

The Committee on Military Nutrition Research (CMNR) has reviewed many studies over the past 10 years on the relationship of nutrition to performance in all aspects of life—both on the job and during relaxation. Food is provided for military personnel on the military bases through garrison dining facilities and during field operations through a variety of military operational rations. In garrison, soldiers can choose to eat in the military dining halls, eat at home with their families, or eat in restaurants similar to the American civilian population. In the field, food selection is limited to the operational ration available during the mission. The nutrient level in military food—whether offered in military dining halls or packaged in military operational rations—is guided by the joint Tri-Services Regulation, AR 40-25 (1985). This regulation includes nutritional allowances and standards for active military personnel (the Military Recommended Dietary Allowances [MRDAs]), nutrient standards for operational and restricted rations (for example, survival rations), military menu guidance, and a chapter on nutrition education. The MRDAs are based on the Recommended Dietary Allowances (RDAs) developed by the FNB to provide for the basic nutritional needs of all healthy Americans (NRC, 1989b). The military operational rations are thus designed to provide a healthy diet for military personnel that includes additional energy and nutrients as may be needed to perform heavy work or meet the demands of environmental extremes.

Unfortunately, in training and field operations, military personnel often do not eat their rations in amounts adequate to meet energy expenditures. Consequently, they lose weight and potentially risk loss of effectiveness both in physical and cognitive performance. The U.S. Army's concern about potential

9

performance degradation has led to a consideration of the cause of this underconsumption in the field.

In March 1993, the CMNR was asked to assist a collaborative program between scientists at the U.S. Army Research Institute of Environmental Medicine (USARIEM) and the U.S. Army Natick Research, Development and Engineering Center (NRDEC, who develop food products and test their acceptability) by reviewing recent research in military settings that addresses these issues, coupled with more general research on the effects of the following on food intake: physiology (hydrations status, biological rhythms), the food itself (quality, quantity, variety, learned preferences, food expectations), food packaging and marketing, and social factors (the eating situation, food appropriateness, social facilitation and inhibition). The purpose was to (1) evaluate whether the consistent energy deficit recorded in military personnel in field settings could significantly affect performance and (2) discuss potential strategies that could be used by the military to reduce underconsumption.

The CMNR was asked to consider the results from military research and from the other studies and also to address the following five questions posed by the Army about soldier underconsumption.

1. Why do soldiers underconsume (not meet energy expenditure needs) in field operations?

2. What factors influence underconsumption in field operations? Identify the relative importance of rations, environment, eating situation, and the individual.

3. At what level of underconsumption is there a negative impact on physical or cognitive performance?

4. Given the environment of military operations, what steps are suggested to enhance ration consumption? To overcome deficits in food intake? To overcome any degradation in physical or cognitive performance?

5. What further research needs to be done in these areas?

The committee was aware of the complexity of the issue, in particular the question of when a reduction in intake of rations becomes detrimental and can be labeled underconsumption, and at what point undernutrition leads to a decrement in performance. The CMNR decided that the best way to review the state of knowledge in this disparate area was through a workshop at which knowledgeable researchers could review published research with the committee. The workshop therefore was convened on November 3–4, 1993 to assist the CMNR in responding to the Army and provide background information useful for developing its report.

The committee's report, *Not Eating Enough, Overcoming Underconsumption of Military Operational Rations* (IOM, 1995a), provides responses to the five questions the CMNR was asked to address and includes conclusions and recommendations, as well as recommendations for future research. The report also includes the 20 invited papers presented at the workshop.

CONCLUSIONS AND RECOMMENDATIONS

On the basis of the workshop presentations and subsequent discussion by the committee in executive session, the committee concluded that underconsumption in the field may affect the performance of military personnel, particularly if it is associated with rapid weight loss (in excess of 2 lb/wk) in lean, fit individuals with little body fat. Rapid redeployment of troops may not permit regaining lost weight between missions.

Since the goal of field feeding is to provide sufficient water, food energy, and nutrients to maintain the soldier's hydration status, body weight, and lean body mass, the committee recommended that a *field feeding doctrine* should be crafted that incorporates the types and amounts of food offered, issues related to environmental extremes, and actions to be taken with excessive weight loss in the field. From a policy standpoint, the risks that energy deficits will be compounded by uncontrollable events in combat are considerable, and thus any consumption deficits are undesirable. The guiding principle of this field feeding doctrine is that the energy intakes of military personnel during training and combat operations should be adequate to meet their energy expenditures. The level of individual body weight loss should determine the actions to be taken.

While underconsumption of operational rations in the training environment is not likely to result in significant reduction in physical or cognitive performance, it may be indicative of a more severe problem when soldiers are under the extreme stresses of impending or actual combat. Therefore steps to minimize underconsumption in training environments may be important when the stress of actual combat operations are imposed.

Additionally, the CMNR recommends the following:

• Ensure that energy intakes match energy expenditures
• Keep soldiers well-hydrated to avoid a decline in appetite due to dehydration.
• Continue efforts to enhance all military rations.
• Provide guidance to commanders regarding the effects of underconsumption on performance and how to minimize the adverse effects of the field environment on food intake.

AREAS FOR FUTURE RESEARCH

The information in this report is primarily derived from data collected during field training exercises. While these observations are important, the impact of the actual exposure to the stresses of combat or impending hostile action is certainly likely to be much greater. Carefully evaluated feedback from soldiers who were deployed in operations such as Vietnam, Desert Storm, and possibly Somalia and Panama could add further insight and realism to the possible extent of underconsumption and influencing factors (e.g., the degree of anxiety, fear, and climatic condition) that would go beyond the information obtained in training exercises. Acquiring information on the coping mechanism used by soldiers under these conditions may be useful in considering how to overcome these problems and suggest important areas for research.

The CMNR recognizes the concern that the loss of weight by personnel during training and operations poses to the military. The scientists at USARIEM and NRDEC have conscientiously followed this issue and conducted carefully planned research programs that have evaluated the impact of food-intake patterns on performance and the factors influencing food intake. The committee made suggestions for future areas of study that would build on this excellent research base.

The committee also commends the development of Kitchen Company Level Field Feeding-Enhanced (KCLFF-E) equipment and the concept of having cooks forward with combat units. After implementation, this system requires follow-up evaluation as to its effectiveness and ways it can be improved.

* * * * *

The full conclusions and recommendations from this report are included in Appendix C.

A Review of the Revision of the Medical Services Nutrition Allowances, Standards, and Education (AR 40-25, 1985)

In 1990, the Department of the Army began to discuss the need to revise the current version of the Military Recommended Dietary Allowances (MRDAs, AR 40-25, 1985). COL Eldon W. Askew, Ph.D., (former) Chief, Military Nutrition Division (currently the Military Nutrition and Biochemistry Division), U.S. Army Research Institute of Environmental Medicine (USARIEM) requested that the Committee on Military Nutrition Research (CMNR) discuss the MRDA review and revision. The committee's role was to evaluate, comment upon, and make specific recommendations regarding changes in the MRDAs designed to reflect changes where appropriate, in the latest version of the Recommended Dietary Allowances (RDAs) (NRC, 1989b) and other relevant national policy statements on nutrition and health, such as the Surgeon General's Report on Nutrition and Health (DHHS, 1988) and *Diet and Health: Implications for Reducing Chronic Disease Risk* (NRC, 1989a).

In November 1990, the committee heard an historical overview of military involvement with dietary recommendations and presentations on the feasibility of attaining governmentally-established dietary recommendations and the process of establishing RDAs. The committee then began an in-depth discussion of the concerns related to the revision of the MRDA; however, the committee deferred further discussion and formulation of recommendations because the Army was in the process of drafting a revised MRDA.

In 1993 the committee received a draft of the MRDAs for review and comment. A subcommittee of the CMNR reviewed the comparison document and the original and draft revisions in detail. The subcommittee found a number

13

of aspects of the revised draft confusing and discussed their findings with the full committee. The CMNR concluded that the confusion generated by the present draft could most likely be alleviated through expansion of several sections and the addition of explanatory footnotes and text. The committee verbally conveyed a request for additional materials to Office of the Surgeon General, Department of the Army (OTSG, DA) and deferred further discussion and formulation of recommendations until receipt of additional material or a second revised draft.

In late January 1994, the CMNR received another revision of the MRDAs for their consideration and recommendations. The committee included discussion of this revision in their executive session after a workshop in February 1994. After the initiation of the current grant in November 1994, the completion of this letter report (along with other outstanding commitments from the previous grant) was a priority for the committee. The completed report was delivered in October 1995. The letter report is thus based on past reviews of AR 40-25, reviews of military rations and ration developments, workshops on nutrient requirements for military personnel in environmental extremes, and committee deliberations regarding the present version, and is a thoughtfully developed presentation incorporating the scientific opinion of the CMNR and comments of the anonymous peer review panel of the National Research Council.

CONCLUSIONS AND RECOMMENDATIONS

It is the view of the CMNR that there does not appear to be a scientific basis to have distinct military recommended dietary allowances for individuals performing duties in normal peacetime military operations and non-field conditions. However, since the MRDAs have an extensive history of use by the military in areas such as menu planning and procurement of military rations, the committee recognizes that they may serve an essential purpose beyond that usually identified with the RDAs. In addition, nutritional standards for the development and procurement of operational and restricted rations are necessary to assure that the issued rations meet the needs of service men and women whose entire diet while under simulated or actual combat conditions may consist of the issued rations for extended periods of time, such as experienced during Operation Desert Shield/Storm and during peace-keeping operations in Somalia and Haiti.

The staffs of OTSG, DA and U.S. Army Medical Research and Materiel Command are urged to review whether there continues to be a need to maintain separate MRDAs in light of existing information that has been developed by the Institute of Medicine, U.S. Department of Health and Human Services, and other organizations for the general population.

The CMNR recommends that the table on nutritional standards for operational and restricted rations be retained and that the narrative accompanying the table values explain clearly how the reference values were derived.

If it is determined by the OTSG, DA that the military version of the RDAs is to be maintained, the CMNR recommends that serious consideration be given to the future mechanism for development of these sections as well as the nutrient standards for operational or restricted rations. The CMNR cannot identify a group within the existing Department of Defense structure with a sufficient depth and breadth of expertise to develop these recommendations. There is a critical need for a group of individuals who are familiar with the development of RDAs to assist in the derivation of the MRDAs as well as the nutritional standards.

The CMNR further recommends that, if it continues to be the view of the OTSG, DA that the MRDAs and nutritional standards for operational and restricted rations are needed, then:

• the scientific expertise at USARIEM should be involved in the future in the development of such standards to assure consideration of the findings of research conducted by the Military Nutrition Division at USARIEM;

• a joint review by nutritionists/dietitians from each of the services is desirable to assure consideration of issues of special concern to each of the branches of the military, in the development of these MRDAs and standards since they are applicable to the Army, Air Force, and Navy; and

• timely consideration by the military of dietary recommendations developed by the Food and Nutrition Board should occur as new versions are released.

* * * * *

The full text of this letter report is included as Appendix D.

A Review of Issues Related to Iron Status in Women During U.S. Army Basic Combat Training

At a planning meeting on October 30, 1995, the Committee on Military Nutrition Research (CMNR) was asked by the Military Nutrition Division (MND, currently the Military Nutrition and Biochemistry Division), U.S. Army Research Institute of Environmental Medicine (USARIEM) and the U.S. Army Medical Research and Materiel Command (USAMRMC) to provide additional scientific guidance to the MND staff in reviewing their recent research related to iron deficiency in military women during U.S. Army Basic Combat Training (BCT). The committee's task was to review the previously published Army technical reports and new material presented at the subsequent meeting on November 13, 1995. The committee was asked to evaluate, comment upon, and make specific recommendations regarding these studies and proposed research plans, as well as to write a formal report that included responses to the following nine questions:

1. Do the data from recent research studies indicate that there is a problem related to iron deficiency in Army women in BCT?
2. Do the data indicate that the incidence of iron deficiency or low iron stores among military women is different from what exists in women with the same demographic characteristics in the civilian population?
3. In terms of military readiness, would military women benefit from a nutritional intervention?
4. Are there additional medical considerations related to iron status in military women that need to be addressed?
5. Should there be periodic screening of military women for anemia or iron deficiency?

17

6. In military personnel with low iron stores as well as anemia, is there an impairment of military readiness that is gender specific?

7. Are there additional analyses that should be conducted with the data in Friedl et al. (1990), Klicka et al. (1993), Westphal et al. (1995), or Westphal et al. (draft manuscript, 1995) on iron status issues in women in BCT? For future studies, are there additional specific analyses that should be considered?

8. What are the CMNR recommendations regarding the proposed intervention study?

9. Emphasis of the meeting on November 13, 1995 was on data collected during BCT, should there be additional research with military women dealing with iron status in military women in general?

To assist the CMNR in developing responses to these questions, John L. Beard, Department of Nutrition, The Pennsylvania State University, University Park, and Sean Lynch, Hematology and Oncology, Veterans Administration Medical Center, Hampton, Virginia, served as special consultants, who participated in the meeting and the initial discussion with the committee regarding this report. The report was drafted by the CMNR in executive session on the day following the meeting and was delivered to the sponsor in December 1995. It is a thoughtfully developed presentation incorporating the scientific opinion of the CMNR and the comments of the anonymous peer review panel of the National Research Council.

CONCLUSIONS

It is the view of the CMNR that iron status is an important issue for military women. From the preliminary data presented at this meeting, the potential for some compromise in physical performance has been demonstrated with low iron stores. Of equal military concern are the possible effects on cognitive performance that may result from impaired iron nutrition. Therefore, additional research should be conducted on the most susceptible groups of military women. It is important to determine whether the compromised iron status observed in women in BCT affects performance; therefore, initial studies should emphasize this issue, using an iron supplement that has the greatest potential for preventing or correcting decrements in iron status with appropriate nutrition counseling stressing the importance of taking such supplements, to help assure compliance with the study design. Following this determination, it then will be important to determine whether appropriate nutrition education methods can achieve similar results.

Since the stresses of military training are an approximation of the anticipated stresses of actual combat, it is important to collect and evaluate broadly all pertinent information from women involved in rigorous, physically stressful military training.

Any analysis of iron status must take into consideration the possible presence of any concurrent infectious or inflammatory processes, which are known to affect rapidly the results of clinical laboratory parameters used to measure iron status.

RECOMMENDATIONS

• Intervention studies be conducted with women in BCT to identify cognitive and physical performance decrements that may be related to iron status.

• An evaluation of the most appropriate approaches to correcting deficits in iron status be made (i.e., nutrition education versus iron supplements).

• An analysis of existing data be conducted using models of iron deficiency previously recommended for the NHANES II and III studies.

• A screening program for military women be established to identify the extent of deficits in iron status and periods of greatest vulnerability, in order that remedial steps can be instituted where appropriate.

• Enlistment of any individual with iron deficiency anemia be delayed until this medically-reversible condition has been corrected.

FUTURE RESEARCH CONSIDERATIONS

• Evaluate the effectiveness of dietary intervention using nutrition education in maintaining iron status.

• Evaluate the impact of dieting measures to meet weight standards on iron status and the potential for nutrition educational approaches to assist women in maintaining iron status when restricting calorie consumption.

• If a relationship between iron status and physical and cognitive performance is found, determine the measure of iron deficiency that best correlates with performance and the extent of iron deficiency that results in a compromised performance.

• In conjunction with monitoring iron status of military women, survey the impact of iron (and other macro- and micronutrient) status on immune function and the impact of iron status on the cardiovascular and pulmonary systems.

• If studies confirm instances of compromised iron status (in individuals who are free of active infections or inflammatory processes), evaluate various delivery systems to minimize or eliminate deficits in iron status such as:

    – a diet naturally high in iron (along with nutrition education), and
    – periodic nutritional supplements of iron (e.g., daily, weekly) (following a review of the dosage and effectiveness [as well as risk of complications such as gastrointestinal side-effects] as reported in the scientific literature).

• If such delivery systems prove to be ineffective, consider the evaluation of other interventions, such as:

    − iron delivered orally in a hydrodynamically balanced solution (Cook et al., 1990), and
    − the safety and effectiveness of oral heme iron.

* * * * *

The full text of this letter report plus the responses to the questions are included in Appendix E.

Nutritional Needs in Cold and in High-Altitude Environments

Military operations are frequently conducted in locations where soldiers are exposed to desert, arctic, and high-altitude environmental extremes. The success of such operations will be influenced by how well humans can perform in these extreme conditions. Gradual adaptation to these environments aids physiological acclimatization. However, military missions rarely can be planned to allow lengthy acclimatization periods. The recent peace-keeping operation in Bosnia is an example of an operation conducted under adverse conditions with little time initially for preparation or acclimatization. Regardless of climatic conditions, troops must be supplied with food, weapons, housing, and other support facilities that will enable the immediate performance of their mission.

Previously, the Committee on Military Nutrition Research (CMNR) was requested by the U.S. Army Research Institute of Environmental Medicine (USARIEM) to provide reviews and recommendations on nutritional needs of soldiers in environmental extremes, such as the parallel review of the previous CMNR report on nutritional needs in hot climates (IOM, 1993a). In 1993, the CMNR was asked by USARIEM to review research pertaining to nutrient requirements for working in cold and in high-altitude terrestrial environments. While there are differences in the stresses imposed by cold as compared to high-altitude environments, there are enough similarities to make them suitable to address concurrently. In addition, the committee was asked to address the increased energy demands of such environments, consider whether these environments elicit an increased requirement for other specific nutrients, interpret these diverse data in terms of military applications, and make recommendations regarding the application of this information to military operational rations.

Committee members decided that the best way to review the state of knowledge in this diverse area was through a small workshop at which knowledgeable researchers could review published research and provide an update on current knowledge, and a subgroup of the CMNR met in August 1993 to identify the key topics for review and the speakers with expertise in these topics. The workshop was convened on January 31 to February 1, 1994 and included presentations from individuals familiar with or having expertise in cold and in high-altitude topics, as well as from military commanders familiar with working and training personnel in these environments. Speakers were asked to provide reviews of their area of expertise, which in turn assisted the committee in responding to a series of 15 questions, which have been summarized into the following two overriding questions:

1. Aside from increased energy demands, do cold or high-altitude environments elicit an increased demand or requirement for specific nutrients?
2. Can performance be enhanced in cold or high-altitude environments by the provision of increased amounts of specific nutrients?

On the day after the workshop, the CMNR met in executive session to review the issues and draw some tentative conclusions. Committee members subsequently met in a series of working sessions to draft the summary and recommendations. The committee's report, *Nutritional Needs in Cold and in High-Altitude Environments, Applications for Military Personnel in Field Operations* (IOM, 1996a), was originally released in March 1996 as a preliminary report in response to troop deployment to Bosnia, and in May 1996, the full report, including 22 papers presented at the workshop, was released.

CONCLUSIONS

The energy requirement for work both in the cold and at high altitudes is increased. However, the increased requirement is adequately met by the cold weather operational rations currently in use. Energy in these rations is primarily provided in the form of carbohydrate. There is insufficient evidence at this time to support providing an increased amount of any specific nutrient in the cold or at high altitudes beyond that already provided in current operational rations.

Additionally, the CMNR emphasizes the critical importance of water discipline, availability of safe fluids for drinking, and a clear understanding on the part of all troops involved in operations or training in cold and in high-altitude environments of the importance of maintaining fluid intake. An impressive body of evidence has already been generated to define the nutritional needs of troops required to engage in military operations under environmental conditions of extreme cold and/or high altitudes.

RECOMMENDATIONS AND AREAS FOR FUTURE RESEARCH

The committee's extensive list of recommendations and areas for future research can be summarized as follows:

To Commanders:
• Ensure adequate ration consumption.
• Provide high-energy, high-carbohydrate rations. When necessary, adjust rations to provide up to 40 percent of their calories in the form of calorie-dense fat to ensure an adequate supply of food energy in a form that can be quickly consumed.
• Enforce the adequate consumption of fluids through training similar to hot climates.
• Redeploy only those who have regained body mass or weight lost in prior field operations. Provide education regarding the physiological changes and symptoms of altitude-related illnesses.

To Researchers:
• Investigate the potential benefits of supplemental antioxidants, for example vitamin E, in preventing the oxidative damage that may result from work at high altitudes.
• Determine the optimum intake of micronutrients and whether micronutrient supplements will improve performance.
• Evaluate the effect of providing diet-related pharmaceutical compounds, such as caffeine and tyrosine, on the decline in cognitive function that accompanies exposure to adverse environmental conditions.

Additionally, the committee believes that the military services, through volunteer participation in studies and surveys, offer an excellent and often unique opportunity to generate research data and statistics on the nutrition, health, and well-being of service personnel. It is important that future studies include men and women representative of the full range of ages in the active duty military. These findings can be directly applied to improve both the health of military personnel and that of the general U.S. population.

* * * * *

The full conclusions and recommendations from this report are included in Appendix F.

Pennington Biomedical Research Center September 1996 Site Visit

Congress mandated in the 1988 Department of Defense (DoD) appropriations bill that $3.5 million be allocated over 3 years by the Army to fund research programs at Louisiana State University's Pennington Biomedical Research Center (PBRC). Support for the PBRC was continued in 1992 with a 5-year, $13 million grant to conduct "Military Nutrition Research: Six Tasks to Address Medical Factors Limiting Soldier Effectiveness."

The staff at the U.S. Army Research Institute of Environmental Medicine (USARIEM), in consultation with the Committee on Military Nutrition Research (CMNR), periodically reviews and makes recommendations on research projects proposed by the PBRC. In June 1989 the CMNR was first asked to review the research plans of the PBRC funded through the DoD appropriations and submitted a letter report with its recommendations to the Army (IOM, 1989). In September 1991 as the initial 3-year grant to the PBRC was nearing completion, the CMNR was asked to review the progress of the PBRC, which resulted in a letter report that was submitted to the Army in May 1992 (IOM, 1992c). The CMNR again visited the PBRC in June 1992 to review new research plans as proposed by the PBRC for a renewal of their contract with the Army. The committee focused its attention on the areas of neuroscience and menu modification, and these reviews were transmitted as reports in May and December 1992 (IOM, 1992c,d).

At the request of Harris R. Lieberman, Military Nutrition and Biochemical Division, USARIEM, members of the CMNR met at the PBRC in Baton Rouge, Louisiana on September 18–20, 1996. The purpose of this meeting was to review and evaluate the progress on work related to the U.S. Army grant to the PBRC, "Military Nutrition Research: Six Tasks to Address Medical Factors Limiting Soldier Effectiveness," and to hear proposals for research to be initiated under the new appropriation of the Pennington military nutrition research program.

Prior to the meeting, the CMNR reviewed: (1) the preproposal requesting funding for the continuation of the agreement between PBRC and USARIEM for 5 years beginning April 1, 1997 for military nutrition studies at the PBRC and background materials; (2) the Pennington Biomedical Research Center Annual Reports for 1991 and 1996 submitted by the principal investigator Donna H. Ryan to the Army; and (3) past CMNR reviews of PBRC activities in the form of letter reports.

The Committee on Military Nutrition Research's activity during this site visit included (1) hearing presentations by PBRC staff members on the progress of current research efforts and proposals for research to be initiated under the new appropriation to the PBRC military nutrition research program; (2) discussing the progress and proposals in a closed session of CMNR members with the Army sponsor; (3) evaluating the progress and proposed activity in an executive session of committee members; and (4) developing a brief report to the Army stating the committee's conclusions and recommendations.

Subsequent to approval of the final draft by the CMNR, this report was reviewed in confidence by a separate anonymous scientific review group. The CMNR evaluated the anonymous comments of these reviewers and incorporated their suggestions where appropriate. This report is thus a thoughtfully developed presentation that incorporates the scientific opinion of the Committee on Military Nutrition Research and the anonymous National Research Council reviewers.

OVERALL CONCLUSIONS AND RECOMMENDATIONS

• The committee finds that the Clinical Research Laboratory is vital to the PBRC and to USARIEM. The availability of this laboratory to USARIEM has, in large measure, solved a critical need that existed for some time prior to 1990 to obtain timely and accurate analytical support for field studies on the nutritional status of military personnel and for the evaluation of military rations designed to meet their needs.

• Of concern to the committee is the lower than expected rate of publication in the scientific literature of the data produced for USARIEM by the PBRC.

• The committee recommends continued support for and integration of the Clinical Research Laboratory, Stable Isotope Laboratory, Menu Modification/Enhancing Military Diets Project, and Nutrient Database Integration Laboratory at a level consistent with USARIEM needs. Experimental studies utilizing the technique of doubly labeled water as well as the incorporation of studies within the Metabolic Units Project employing isotopes to evaluate nutrient utilization should receive high priority in developing projects of interest to the Army.

• The committee recommends that additional collaborations be sought for the incorporation of the most current laboratory methodologies for nutrient analysis, with restriction of effort to obtaining data that are not currently available or are extrapolated.

• The committee recommends that additional expenditure of resources be permitted for collaboration on development and evaluation of various clinical laboratory tests to assess immune function.

• The committee recommends the use of human subjects in metabolic studies that will be more inclusive and better directed to the needs of the military.

• The committee believes that with expert consultation and with the development of an appropriate animal model to evaluate the impact of stress on brain function, the Stress, Nutrition, and Work Performance project can contribute much in the way of basic studies in support of the military mission. On the other hand, the committee does not feel that continuing the development of clinical studies on sleep deprivation in the Sleep Laboratory is of particular value to the Army.

• The committee finds that the Menu Modification/Enhancing Military Diets Project as well as the Nutrient Database Integration Laboratory are valuable to the Army mission and provide needed support to USARIEM. Additional efforts with regard to nutrition education should be incorporated in order to meet Military Dietary Goals.

• The committee recommends integrating the proposed new projects, "Stress, Nutrition, and Work Performance" and "Stress, Nutrition and Immune Function," in both the basic laboratory studies and the clinical studies; they can provide a high degree of military relevance and should be strongly supported. Whenever possible and as appropriate, human subjects should be utilized rather than animal models in these project areas.

* * * * *

The committee's review of the PBRC's military nutrition research program, along with conclusions and recommendations, are included in Appendix G.

Emerging Technologies for Nutrition Research

As the U.S. military faces the twenty-first century, it must contend with changes in the nature of warfare and deployment that have significant implications for individual performance. The more frequent redeployment of soldiers (necessitated by downsizing and by changing military strategies) mandates greater concern for their physical health and well-being and, therefore, the development of cutting-edge techniques for field assessment of health and nutritional status. Such assessment tools must demonstrate reproducibility and reliability in field tests, must be noninvasive, and must cause minimal interference with battlefield operations. Reliance upon techniques that are tied to laboratories must give way to ambulatory assessment. Budgetary constraints, coupled with the need to stay at the forefront of research, dictate that careful consideration be given to identifying the best available and emerging technologies and making priority decisions regarding which ones should be undertaken directly by the military, which deserve investment of funds to foster military applications, and which are best left to the private sector.

In 1994, the Committee on Military Nutrition Research (CMNR) was asked by the scientists at the U.S. Army Research Institute of Environmental Medicine (USARIEM) to identify and evaluate new technologies to determine whether the technologies will provide useful tools to help solve important issues in military nutrition research in the areas identified by USARIEM. The committee was requested: (1) to provide a survey of newly available and emerging techniques for the assessment and optimization of nutritional and physiological status and performance, and (2) to evaluate the potential of these techniques to contribute to future research efforts involving military personnel. In addition, the committee was asked to make recommendations regarding the practicality and the applica-

29

tion of such techniques in field settings and to include in its response the answers to the following six questions:

1. Will the technologies be a significant improvement over current technologies?
2. How likely are the technologies to mature sufficiently for practical use?
3. What is the cost/benefit ratio of the new technologies, and how expensive (in both monetary and personnel terms) will they be to employ compared with the importance of the information they will provide?
4. Are the technologies of such critical value that their development should be supported by Department of Defense funds—such as can be provided by the Small Business Innovative Research program?
5. How practical are the technologies? Will they require dedicated personnel and complex, exotic equipment? Will the data provided be difficult to analyze?
6. Can the technologies be used in the field (could they be used in the field or used to analyze samples collected in the field)?

Recognizing that there were a large number of technologies that could be reviewed and the need to limit the scope of this review to those areas of most interest to USARIEM, six relevant research areas for review were identified, with the primary criterion for inclusion being the possibility for application to field research: body composition, tracer techniques to evaluate metabolism and energy expenditure, ambulatory methods to determine energy expenditure, molecular and cellular approaches to nutrition and immune function, and functional and behavioral measures of nutritional status. To assist the CMNR in responding to the questions, a workshop was convened on May 22–23, 1995, in Washington, D.C., that included presentations from individuals with expertise in the aforementioned areas.

Committee members subsequently met with staff several times over the course of a year and a half and worked separately and together using the authored papers, additional reference materials provided by the staff, and personal expertise and experience with the methods to draft the overview, summary, conclusions, and recommendations, which were reviewed by an anonymous panel of peers according to National Research Council policy.

This report, *Emerging Technologies for Nutrition Research: Potential for Assessing Military Performance Capability* (IOM, 1997), looks at newer technologies that are being employed to identify and study basic issues that may be significant in nutrition research, with evaluation being limited to technologies discussed at the workshop. It provides responses to the questions posed to the CMNR, conclusions, and recommendations, as well 24 invited papers presented at the workshop.

CONCLUSIONS

- Methods of measuring body composition are relevant and important to the military to assure accuracy and fairness in the application of body composition measures to accession and retention of military personnel.
- Anthropometric measures are the most applicable methods for evaluating compliance with military standards of body fat. The more sophisticated technologies of computerized axial tomography scanning, magnetic resonance imaging (MRI), and dual-energy x-ray absorptiometry (DXA) are useful tools for developing application equations from anthropometric measures to estimate body fat.
- Bioelectrical impedance analysis is a less-reliable method of measuring body fat, but the methodology may be useful in answering specific questions concerning hydration state and function of cell membranes.
- Tracer methodology, particularly the use of stable isotopes, is an important technology for understanding and measuring metabolic processes (the doubly labeled water technique currently is used in studies of energy expenditure in the field and is a cost-effective technology for this purpose). Stable isotopes that can be administered and measured noninvasively through easily obtained samples offer important opportunities to estimate metabolic processes in the field. Central analysis of samples increases the practicality of their use in field studies.
- Ambulatory monitoring techniques, such as the foot strike measurement, also show good promise as field measures of work and energy expenditure.
- The various molecular and cellular technologies are interesting as research methods but are strictly laboratory research tools at present. Observing the development of these techniques and their application will be important for USARIEM, but investing in their in-house development is not recommended at this time. Studies of immune function are potentially very important to the military. An understanding of the effect of the various stresses of military operations on the body's immune function and how these may be modified to aid soldier performance is an important area for investigation.
- The development of vaccines against various infectious diseases of unique significance to the military population but not necessarily of significance to the civilian population may be very important in sustaining the ability of the soldier to operate effectively in the field. Oral vaccines may be most effective as they tend to mimic the route of exposure to the infectious agents that cause problems in the field.
- The development and production of human antibodies by transgenic plants create dramatic new possibilities for short-term (weeks-to-months) prophylaxis, or therapy, of unusual infectious diseases or toxemias of potential military importance and for which no other forms of immunization currently are available.

• The ability to study the cognitive function of individuals while they perform their duties has great potential for improving soldier performance under stress. Current developments in computerized and miniaturized technology appear to permit expanded studies of real-time cognitive behavior. Support for the development of specific monitoring devices that are compatible with military field equipment may be necessary to implement this technology.

RECOMMENDATIONS

• Anthropometric equations remain the most practical tools for assessment of body composition in field situations. More sophisticated technologies such as DXA and MRI should be used to develop criterion measures for refinement of the equations.

• Tracer methodology is important for measuring energy expenditure and metabolism. Further development of stable isotope techniques in collaboration with the private sector is recommended for greater field applicability.

• A foot-contact method shows promise for ambulatory monitoring of energy expenditure.

• The military should keep abreast of research in the private sector that uses molecular cloning techniques to study the effects of nutritional and other stressors on gene expression, but this research should not be undertaken by the military at this time.

• Development of vaccines that are effective against infectious diseases of unique significance to military populations should be pursued.

• Noninvasive techniques for the assessment of cognitive function during operational task performance should be developed further.

* * * * *

The committee's responses to the questions, conclusions, and recommendations from this report are included in Appendix H.

Assessing Readiness in
Military Women

U.S. military personnel are required to adhere to standards of body composition, fitness, and appearance for the purpose of achieving and maintaining readiness. Military readiness, while encompassing many factors, can be defined briefly as maintenance of optimum health and performance so that deployment can occur at any moment.

In 1992, the Committee on Military Nutrition Research was asked by the U.S. Army to evaluate the body composition and fitness standards for personnel accession and retention in all branches of active service, with regard to the impact of these standards on recruitment, physical fitness, and task performance in the Armed Forces. After conducting a workshop to investigate these issues, the CMNR released a report concluding that the standards of body composition required for women to achieve the desired appearance goal (low fat-free mass [FFM] and percent body fat) seemed to conflict with those necessary for performance of many types of military tasks (higher FFM often accompanied by increased body fat) (IOM, 1992a). The committee recommended that body composition standards be based primarily on considerations of task performance and health and that they be validated with regard to the ethnic diversity of the military population. In addition, the committee recommended the development of task-specific performance tests; development of objective appearance standards, if these were deemed necessary; and continuation of research on the relationships among body composition, health, and physical performance of military personnel. Also recommended was evaluation of the long-term outcome of individuals referred to military weight management programs for failure to adhere to standards.

At the autumn 1994 conference of the Defense Advisory Committee for Women in the Service (DACOWITS), one of the concerns identified by the group was the need to address the body composition and physical fitness

33

standards of the military and the impact of these standards on the health of women, particularly with regard to the potential influence of the standards on food intake and nutritional status. A report, released by the IOM in 1995, which provided recommendations for research on the health of military women identified a number of gaps in research pertaining to the health and performance of military women. These included research on optimal physical fitness for military women, injury prevention, and ways to achieve and assess physical fitness, as well as fitness standards, including those for fitness during pregnancy and the postpartum period.

In 1995, in light of efforts to consider creation of DoD-wide fitness and body composition standards, calls to ensure that all personnel are physically able to perform their assigned tasks, and evidence suggesting that attempts to adhere to body composition and appearance standards may place active-duty women at special risk for inadequate nutrient intake, the CMNR was asked to appoint a subcommittee to examine issues of body composition, fitness, and appearance standards and their impact on the health, nutritional status, and performance of active-duty military women. Specifically, they were asked by the Army to address the following questions:

1. What body composition standards best serve military women's health and fitness, with respect to minimum lean body mass, maximum body fat, and site specificity of fat deposition? Are the appearance goals of the military in conflict with military readiness?

2. Should any part of the Military Recommended Dietary Allowances (MRDAs) be further adjusted for women? Should there be any intervention for active-duty women with respect to food provided, dietary supplementation, or education?

3. What special guidance should be offered with respect to return-to-duty standards and nutrition for women who are pregnant or breastfeeding?

In April 1996, the CMNR convened a subcommittee comprising experts in the areas of body composition, exercise physiology, obesity, women's nutrition, epidemiology and survey design, cognitive psychology, and pregnancy and lactation. Several members of the parent committee were included to provide continuity. The subcommittee was designated the Subcommittee on Body Composition, Nutrition, and Health of Military Women (BCNH).

In considering the questions posed by the military, the subcommittee consulted with a liaison panel composed of military researchers and health care personnel. A workshop was convened in September 1996 to bring together additional military personnel in the areas of physical fitness assessment, training, medicine, and nutrition, as well as civilian researchers and practitioners in the areas of physical fitness and performance, pregnancy, eating disorder assessment, and nutrition.

CONCLUSIONS AND RECOMMENDATIONS

On the basis of the workshop presentations, review of the relevant scientific literature and current military policies the BCNH subcommittee concluded that while the DoD maximum body fat for women is 36 percent, each service sets its own (lower) standards; thus personnel who are out of compliance in their own service may be within the standards of another service. Agreement is poor among results of the service-specific equations used to calculate percent body fat, and in addition, validation of the equations has been called into question because the population used for validation diverges significantly in ethnic profile from that of today's military.

Fitness is assessed by the military coincident with, but independent of, body composition. Data suggests that significant numbers of younger personnel cannot pass the fitness tests. Efforts to show a relationship between body composition and fitness among military women have reached the conclusion that women who are judged to be out of standard with respect to body fat perform better in tests of strength than women who are within the body fat standards. Thus the current body composition assessment procedures may select against retention of those who may be most capable of performing the tasks necessary for military operations while selecting in favor of those who fit an appearance standard.

A summary of the subcommittee's key recommendations are:

• Incorporate the use of body mass index (BMI) and fitness assessment into the current two-tier body composition assessment procedures used to determine compliance with body composition standards (first tier, weight-for-height; second tier, body fat assessment).

• Set the maximum allowable BMI at 25, based on considerations of health and chronic disease, with a maximum body fat of 36 percent if fitness test is passed.

• Develop and validate a single, service-wide, circumferential equation for the assessment of women's body fat.

• Develop task specific, gender-neutral strength and endurance tests and standards for use in the determination of placement in military occupational specialties that require moderate and heavy lifting.

• Encourage military women to achieve and maintain healthy weights through a continuous exercise and fitness program, and provide nutrition education and ongoing counseling if weight loss is a goal.

• Reinforce efforts to provide complete nutritional labeling of all operational ration components and to design ration components that concentrate the nutrients that may be limiting in women's diets.

• Encourage women to engage in a moderate exercise program during pregnancy when medically feasible.

• Set the time allowance for postpartum fitness testing at 180 days, and extend exemption from deployment to 6 months.

• Endorse the 1990 Institute of Medicine guidelines for gestational weight gain, and extend the time allowance for attainment of body weight standards to 1 year when satisfactory progress is being made.

• Redesign surveys to link demographic and personnel information to medical and health information.

* * * * *

The committee's responses to the questions, conclusions, and recommendations from this report are included in Appendix I.

Reducing Stress Fracture in Physically Active Military Women

As part of the Defense Women's Health Research Program, the U.S. Army Medical Research and Materiel Command requested that the Subcommittee on Body Composition, Nutrition, and Health of Military Women (BCNH subcommittee) in addition to their evaluation of the effect of current military fitness and body composition standards on the nutrition and health of military women, also identify and provide recommendations regarding special nutritional considerations of active-duty military women. An area identified for further study in military women concerned the effect of calcium, as well as total energy intake, on the incidence of stress fractures in the short term, and osteoporosis in the long term and the nutrient implications of these conditions.

The incidence of stress fractures during U.S. military basic training is significantly higher in female recruits than in male recruits (IOM, 1992a; 1998a). This injury has a marked impact on the health of service personnel and imposes a significant financial burden on the military by delaying the training of new recruits. Stress fractures increase the length of training time, program costs, and time to military readiness. In addition, stress fractures, a short-term risk, may share their etiology with the long-term risk of osteoporosis.

In order to address these issues adequately in the short timetable of the proposal, the BCNH, a subcommittee of the Committee on Military Nutrition Research (CMNR), held a workshop December 7-9, 1997. The workshop included experts in the areas of endocrinology, calcium metabolism, bone mineral assessment, sports medicine, and military nutrition to evaluate the effects of diet, genetics, and physical activity on bone mineral and calcium status in young servicewomen. Specifically, the subcommittee (and thus, the speakers) were asked to consider the effects of dietary restriction at the levels observed in military women, combined with the physical demands of basic training, both on short-term bone mineral status (and the

37

immediate risk of stress fracture) and on the long-term risk of osteoporosis. In so doing, the subcommittee was asked to respond to the following five questions:

1. Why is the incidence of stress fractures in military basic training greater for women than for men?

2. What is the relationship of genetics and body composition to bone density and the incidence of stress fractures in women?

3. What are the effects of diet, physical activity, contraceptive use, and other lifestyle factors (smoking and alcohol) on the accrual of peak bone mineral content, incidence of stress fractures, and development of osteoporosis in military women?

4. How do caloric restriction and disordered eating patterns affect hormonal balance and the accrual and maintenance of peak bone mineral content?

5. How can the military best ensure that the dietary intakes of active-duty military women in training and throughout their military careers do not contribute to an increased incidence of stress fractures and osteoporosis?

In considering the questions posed by the military (and as a follow-on activity to the subcommittee's earlier report, Assessing Readiness in Military Women [IOM, 1998]), the subcommittee consulted with a liaison panel comprising military researchers and health care personnel. The BCNH subcommittee met in executive session following the workshop to begin drafting their brief report. The subcommittee met in executive session for an additional writing session and to discuss their conclusions and recommendations on January 27, 1998. Based on information gathered from discussion with the workshop speakers, the military liaison panel and a brief review of the literature on bone metabolism and risk factors for bone health, the subcommittee prepared this brief report, *Reducing Stress Fractures in Physically Active Military Women.* The report was submitted to the sponsor in June, 1998.

CONCLUSIONS

Low initial fitness of recruits appears to be the principal factor in the development of stress fractures during basic training. The basic training period may be insufficient time to achieve the aerobic fitness level required and the musculoskeletal adaptations necessary to avoid injury.

Muscle mass, strength, and resistance to fatigue with cyclic loading (bone stress created by rapid or excessive incremental skeletal muscle contraction and loading forces) play a critical role in the development of stress fracture. The etiology of stress fracture is multifactorial, and bone mineral density is only one contributing factor. Genetics and body mass, specifically muscle mass, are also important determinants of stress fracture.

Energy intake by military women should be adequate to maintain weight during training. Nutritional modification of diets of incoming recruits cannot effectively prevent stress fractures during the short term of basic training. The use of oral contraceptives is not contraindicated. Exogenous estrogen-progestagen hormones may positively affect peak bone mass reached in adulthood whereas any conditions that induce estrogen deficiency (e.g. training regimen, diet, weight loss) may adversely affect the skeleton. It is likely that maintenance of appropriate body weight is important in preventing the onset of secondary amenorrhea.

RECOMMENDATIONS

The subcommittee's key recommendations and recommendations for future research are summarized as follows:

Training and Physical Fitness Assessment
• Develop a more appropriate fitness standard for women through a structured program prior to basic training or through an integrated program with basic training. This program should be designed to increase the level of activity gradually.
• Focus the basic training program on alternating low impact loading and higher impact routines that lead to cardiopulmonary fitness to avoid training errors.
• Emphasize a program of continual physical fitness; this will assist in the maintenance of weight, fat-free mass, and bone mass in all servicemembers.
• Perform fitness and body composition assessments more frequently, and in a manner that will foster adherence to healthy weight and physical fitness practices.
• Use of bone mineral measurements for routine screening of recruits to determine stress fracture susceptibility is not recommended at this time.
• Develop a research effort to compile data from all military services on initial fitness level of recruits by age, gender, and race/ethnicity
• Develop a research effort to collect stress fracture incidence statistics by age, gender, race/ethnicity, and skeletal site, using a gender-independent, standardized definition and collect data during a comparable time frame from all military services during both the basic training and post-training periods.
• As recommended previously (AFEB, 1996), develop research to determine the types of activities that may predispose women to stress fractures, especially in the pelvic region and upper leg. Develop modifications of these activities in basic training to lower risk.

Nutrition and Related Factors

• Ensure that energy intakes by military women are consistent and adequate to maintain weight during intense physical fitness training.

• Aim aggressive education programs at helping military women identify and select appropriate foods and fortified food products to meet their nutrient requirements.

• Continue to gather dietary intake data and evidence concerning calcium intakes throughout a soldiers' career as training programs, food choices and food supply change over time.

• Develop research efforts to assist in identifying those factors, such as diet, lifestyle, and ethnicity, that may contribute to achieving peak bone mass, as well as components of military programs that may interfere with this process.

• Develop research to assess the effect of military women's dietary energy status on the secretion of hormones that affect bone health, particularly in situations of high stress. Little is known about the prevalence and underlying causes of menstrual cycle disturbances (oligomenorrhea, amenorrhea).

• Evidence indicates that oral contraceptives have no detrimental effects on bone mineral density, and may in fact have a positive effect. Develop a research program to determine the effects of implant and injectable contraceptives on bone mineral density and bone health.

* * * * *

The committee's responses to the questions, conclusions, and recommendations from this report are included in Appendix J.

A Review of Antioxidants and Oxidative Stress in Military Personnel

The Office of the Surgeon General (OSG), through the U.S. Army Medical Research and Materiel Command (USAMRMC), requested CMNR to provide interim guidance on the potential value of supplemental antioxidants for the health and readiness of service members. The questions posed by the OSG related to the value of specific supplements (Vitamins C, E and β-carotene) administered proactively to protect individuals against hazards in the military environment which may not be typical of exposures in the general U.S. population. To address this issue, the CMNR held a workshop in Washington, D.C. on July 29-31, 1998 and produced a letter report with conclusions, recommendations and responses to the following three key questions:

1. What is the strength of the evidence to suggest that oxidative stress is a concern for service members during extremes of physical activity and other stresses encountered in training and operations?

2. What is the strength of the evidence that vitamin C, vitamin E, and/or β-carotene are likely to protect health and performance of service members exposed to multiple environmental stresses during military training and operations (e.g. severe air pollution in some urban environments; radiation hazards to crew at altitude; radio frequency radiation hazards on ships and around communications facilities; lung and tissue blast overpressure effects and physical and psychological stresses in extreme training courses such as Ranger training and USMC crucible training)?

3. Is there evidence of any health risk associated with supplementing intakes of vitamin C, vitamin E, and β-carotene by service members, with the

intention of maintaining health and performance in adverse military training and operational environments?

CONCLUSIONS

• Information presented at this meeting, in earlier CMNR reports, and other scientific literature provided evidence that military service leads to exposure to unique oxidative stresses that may have adverse health consequences. Some of these stresses are reasonably well characterized, such as those associated with strenuous exercise, work in extremes of environmental temperatures, and at altitude. Much less is known about other sources of oxidative stress, such as radiofrequency and microwave radiation hazards, exposure to blast overpressure, and psychological stress related to extreme training courses or deployment.

• Military rations formulated in accordance with the MRDAs provide nutrients in amounts consistent with meeting nutrient needs—including the antioxidant nutrients—when these rations are consumed at levels required to maintain body weight in the usual range of physical activity for military task requirements. There is little evidence that supplementation with vitamins C, E or with β-carotene in normal conditions (i.e. in garrison) would enhance overall health.

• There is little evidence currently available to indicate that supplementation of vitamins C and E and β-carotene would be beneficial in protecting against short term, acute oxidative stress. In addition, the use of antioxidant compounds to minimize this stress is not without risk.

RECOMMENDATIONS

• Effective methods of promoting lifestyle changes as outlined in *Diet and Health* (NRC, 1989a), *Healthy People 2000* (DHHS, 1991) and *Healthy People 2010* (in draft) should be developed as these have the greatest potential of maintaining health and performance of military personnel and their dependents, particularly in view of the introductory comments of Lt. General Blanck concerning the transition of military medicine to a health promotion emphasis.

• Aggressive educational efforts should be directed to military personnel engaged in operations of various intensities and in stressful environments on the importance of striving to maintain food intakes consistent with physical demands and energy requirements to avoid excessive weight loss.

• Emphasis should be placed on meeting the recommendations of the Dietary Guidelines for Americans (USDA/DHHS, 1995) rather than supplementing with individual nutrients.

• Supplementation should not be considered except in specific high stress situations where intake is likely to be markedly inadequate. If supplementation is determined to be necessary, however, data on the benefits of doses exceeding 100 mg/day of vitamin C and 50 mg/day of vitamin E as alpha tocopherol are not definitive and need to be confirmed. Supplementation of β-carotene for military personnel is **NOT** recommended at this time.

• As study results become available in trials of the interrelationships of vitamin E and vitamin C to muscle soreness and to immunological function, these recommendations should be reviewed again.

FUTURE RESEARCH RECOMMENDATIONS

• Research focused on the protective effects of antioxidants against acute oxidative stress is strongly encouraged as information is most lacking in this area.

• Validation of a battery of biomarkers for detecting oxidative tissue damage in human subjects in ambulatory or field situations.

• Evaluation of the extent to which the presence of tissue oxidative damage impacts performance.

• The extent and duration of oxidative stress that might be associated with hyperoxia, prolonged exposure to ionizing radiation, radiofrequency, blast overpressure, and psychological stress.

• Supplementation of vitamins C, E and ß-carotene in a controlled, randomized way so that their true efficacy in decreasing oxidative tissue damage based on validated biomarkers can be determined. This research is essential both with respect to optimizing health and performance of personnel, and optimizing cost effectiveness.

* * * * *

The full text of the letter report plus the responses to the questions are in Appendix K.

Military Strategies for Sustainment of Nutrition and Immune Function in the Field

The infectious disease threats facing soldiers are multiple and vary with geography. In fact, during major wars, infectious diseases usually have accounted for more noneffective days than combat wounds or nonbattle injuries. Combined stressors may reduce the normal ability of soldiers to resist pathogens, may increase susceptibility to biological agents employed against them, and may reduce effectiveness of vaccines intended to protect them. Studies in multistressor environments, such as basic training and the Special Forces' assessment and selection course, demonstrated that higher energy intakes better sustained indices of immune status (even in the face of other stressors). Regardless of operational stressors, troops must be supplied with high quality foods that will enable them to sustain performance and that will counter an array of immunological impairments caused by a host of unknown stressors.

The request for a review of the role of nutrition in immune function and its application to military operations originated with Army scientists from the U.S. Army Research Institute of Environmental Medicine (USARIEM) and U.S. Army Medical Research and Materiel Command (USAMRMC). In December 1995, a subgroup of the Committee on Military Nutrition Research (CMNR) participated in a series of conference calls with USARIEM, USAMRMC, and CMNR staff to identify the key areas that should be reviewed and to solicit suggestions for participants who were active in the research fields of interest. On May 20–21, 1996, the CMNR convened a workshop with presentations from individuals with expertise in nutrition and immune function. The two days following the workshop, the committee met to review workshop papers, additional literature obtained by staff, and begin drafting their summary and recommendations.

45

Additional writing sessions were held September 18–19, 1996, January 29–30, 1997, and March 13–14, 1997.

The Committee on Military Nutrition Research (CMNR) was tasked with assessing the current state of knowledge about immune function to ascertain how military stresses (including food deprivation) could impact unfavorably upon these functions and to evaluate ongoing research efforts by USARIEM scientists to study immune status in Special Forces troops. The committee was asked to include in their response the answers to the following five questions: The speakers invited to the workshop were also asked to address these questions in their presentations and in their chapters.

1. What are the significant military hazards or operational settings most likely to compromise immune function in soldiers?

2. What methods for assessment of immune function are most appropriate in military nutrition laboratory research and what methods are most appropriate for field research?

3. The proinflammatory cytokines have been proposed to decrease lean body mass, mediate thermoregulatory mechanisms, and increase resistance to infectious disease by reducing metabolic activity in a way that is similar to the reduction seen in malnutrition and other catabolic conditions. Interventions to sustain immune function can alter the actions, nutritional costs, and potential changes in the levels of proinflammatory cytokines. What are the benefits and risks to soldiers of such interventions?

4. What are the important safety and regulatory considerations in the testing and use of nutrients or dietary supplements to sustain immune function under field conditions?

5. Are there areas of investigation for the military nutrition research program that are likely to be fruitful in the sustainment of immune function in stressful conditions? Specifically, is there likely to be enough value added to justify adding to operational rations or including an additional component?

CONCLUSIONS

• Many stressful conditions encountered by military personnel have immunological consequences.

• The military's use of prophylactic immunization provides sufficient benefits beyond risk to warrant continued development.

• Pharmacological agents such as aspirin, ibuprofen, and glucocorticoids, which modulate the effects of cytokines, can be used to minimize signs and symptoms of cytokine-induced acute-phase reactions and the nutrient losses that accompany them.

• Evidence to suggest that the administration of recombinant cytokines can modulate immune function in a desirable manner is limited.

- Field studies must be based on the results of prior experiments conducted in controlled laboratory and clinical settings.
- Total energy intake appears to play the greatest role in nutritional modulation of immune function.
- The nutritional status of soldiers should be optimized prior to deployment,
- Nutrients that appear to play a role in immune function include protein, iron, zinc, copper, and selenium; the B-group vitamins, especially B_6, B_{12}, and folate; vitamin A and its precursor, ß-carotene, vitamins C and E; the amino acids glutamine and arginine; and the polyunsaturated fatty acids.
- The effects of providing supplements of vitamins A, C and E, as well as certain polyunsaturated fatty acids and amino acids, prior to, during, or following infections are virtually unknown in young, healthy adult men.
- Excess iron as well as iron deficiency may compromise immune status.
- Glutamine has demonstrated potential for improving immune function in critical illness, but its usefulness in healthy populations is unknown.
- Risks associated with excess consumption of supplements are much more likely for some nutrients than for others. Toxicity and the potential for nutrient–nutrient interactions must be considered individually.

RECOMMENDATIONS

- Use medically appropriate and directed prophylactic medications and procedures to minimize the adverse effects of infectious agents. However, there appears to be no potential value at this time in administration of cytokines or anti-cytokines to healthy military personnel.
- Vigorous research efforts should be undertaken to create and evaluate militarily relevant oral vaccines.
- Military personnel should maintain good physical fitness via a regular, moderate exercise program as a means of sustaining optimum immune function.
- Use methods to minimize psychological stresses, including training, conditioning, and structured briefing and debriefing.
- In view of the compromised immune function noted in studies of Ranger trainees, individuals who have lost significant lean body mass should not be redeployed until this lean mass is regained.
- Nutritional anemias should be treated prior to deployment and individuals classified as anemic[1] and requiring iron supplements should not be deployed.
- Develop and implement nutrition education programs targeted at high-risk military groups, such as Special Forces troops and female soldiers, to communicate information regarding healthy eating habits and supplement use.

---

[1] Iron deficiency anemia is defined as a serum ferritin concentration of less than 12 ng/ml in combination with a hemoglobin of less than 120 g/L.

• General supplementation of military rations above MRDA levels for the purpose of enhancing immune function is NOT recommended.

• The preferred method of providing supplemental nutrients is through a ration component.

• Gain a better understanding of the prevalence of supplement use and abuse by personnel and make strong recommendations for their appropriate use or nonuse.

• Conduct research to determine the appropriate field measures (see Table S-2) for monitoring nutritionally induced immune responses, particularly the presence of acute-phase reactions and changes in immune function of the type and degree that are likely to occur as a result of the nutritional insults suffered by soldiers in typical deployment situations.

• Carefully design research protocols.

• Increase awareness of and potential military application of findings within the civilian research community regarding nutrition and immune function.

RECOMMENDATIONS FOR FUTURE RESEARCH

• Perform *laboratory-based studies* as recommended previously (IOM, 1997) to determine if an interleukin-6 (IL-6)–creatinine ratio (or some comparable measure) can be measured in single "spot" urine samples as an index of the 24-h excretion of IL-6 and determine if 24-h IL-6 excretion is, in turn, a reliable indicator of acute stress response.

• Develop and *field test* appropriate cytokine markers in urine and blood that are reflective of ongoing acute-phase reactions and of changes in immune status in multistress environments.

• Research conducted on the ability of nutrients to influence immune status should place priority on the antioxidant nutrients β-carotene and vitamins C and E.

• Keep apprised of research being conducted in the civilian sector on immune function in physically active women and consider conducting studies on military women in situations of deployment to augment the findings of civilian studies.

• The influence of iron status on the risk of infection requires further investigation. This is also an area of interest to the civilian medical community.

* * * * *

The committee's responses to the questions, conclusions, and recommendations from this report are included in Appendix L.

The Role of Protein and Amino Acids in Sustaining and Enhancing Performance

As the U.S. military faces the millennium and the changing nature of modern warfare, it must anticipate physical and mental challenges never encountered before. Longer periods of intense physical exertion and possible food deprivation; advanced weaponry requiring maximum attention, precision, and decision-making ability; and greater threats of infection, injury, and exposure to environmental stressors are quickly becoming the reality that soldiers face. Military scientists charged with maintaining and optimizing the health and performance of their personnel are looking to the role that nutrition may play in this process, and have expressed particular interest in the body of current research suggesting the importance of protein and amino acids.

Proteins catalyze virtually all chemical reactions in the body, regulate gene expression, comprise the major structural elements of all cells, regulate the immune system, and form the major constituents of muscle. Individual amino acids, the components of proteins, also serve as neurotransmitters, hormones, and modulators of various physiological processes. Every aspect of physiology involves proteins. The relationships between dietary protein and bodily protein metabolism are a major focus of research. In addition, the influences of genetic factors, hormones, physical activity, injury and infectious processes, and environmental stresses on protein metabolism and protein requirements continue to be explored.

The request for this review originated with scientists at USARIEM who were concerned about the unique nutritional demands placed on soldiers during combat. They were particularly concerned about the role that dietary protein may play in controlling muscle mass and strength, response to injury and infection, and cognitive performance.

49

Several previous CMNR reports have focused on issues of protein nutriture and performance. In 1992, the CMNR noted in an evaluation of Army Ranger training that trainees experienced significant loss of muscle mass during periods of intense physical exertion (IOM, 1992b). A follow-up report (IOM, 1993b) found that increases in energy intake only partially prevented such losses. The report *Food Components to Enhance Performance* (IOM, 1994b) briefly considered the influences of protein and amino acids on physical and cognitive performance and response to stress. The most recent CMNR report, *Military Strategies for Sustainment of Nutrition and Immune Function in the Field* (IOM, 1999), considered the effects of diet, including protein and individual amino acids such as glutamine, on immune response. This report looks further into the many questions regarding the optimal level of protein intake in a high-stress field environment. How to measure protein balance and estimate protein requirements accurately; how these requirements are affected by physical activity, gender, hormonal factors, and stress; and whether muscle function and cognition are influenced by protein intake and by individual amino acids are all active areas of research.

The CMNR decided that the best way to review the state of knowledge in this area was through a workshop. The purpose of this workshop was to bring together leading scientists in the field of protein metabolism to seek their assessment of the current state of knowledge and to determine, based on these assessments, on a careful reading of the literature, and on the expertise of the committee members themselves, whether the recommended intakes of protein or individual amino acids for soldiers should be modified.

In May 1996, CMNR and USARIEM personnel met to frame a series of questions, outline the workshop, and identify qualified speakers. A follow-up planning meeting was held in January 1997 and included several members of the Subcommittee on Body Composition, Nutrition, and Health of Military Women. Invited workshop speakers were asked to prepare a paper for presentation and publication that described the key issues of protein metabolism. USARIEM scientists also participated in the workshop, which resulted in a well-rounded group. At the one-day workshop, held in Washington, D.C. on March 13, 1997, each speaker gave a formal presentation, which was followed by questions and a brief discussion period. The proceedings were tape recorded and professionally transcribed. At the end of each group of presentations, a general discussion of the overall topic was held. Immediately after the workshop, the CMNR met in executive session to review the issues, to draft summaries of the presentations, and to provide responses to the sponsor's task questions. Committee members subsequently met with staff in June 1997 and worked separately and together using the authored papers, additional reference materials provided by the staff through limited literature searches, and personal expertise and experience to draft the overview, summary, conclusions, and recommendations.

The principal questions that the CMNR and BCNH (and in turn, the speakers) were asked to address were:

1. Do protein requirements increase with military operational stressors, including high workload and/or energy deficit?

2. What is the optimal protein content (protein to energy ratio) for standard operational rations and, specifically, is the Military Recommended Dietary Allowance (MRDA) for protein in operational rations (100 g/d for men and 80 g/d for women) appropriate? Is the protein MRDA for women appropriate during pregnancy and lactation?

3. Is there evidence that supplementation with specific amino acids (AA) would optimize military performance (cognitive function) during high workload, psychological stress, and/or energy deficit? (See summaries of speakers) Is there a risk of using specific AA supplements during pregnancy, especially the first trimester (i.e., organogenesis)?

4. Are there gender differences in protein requirements in endurance exercise, and if so, what might their implications be for performance in military operations? What is the evidence, if any, that protein facilitates muscle building?

The committees met after the workshop in executive session, as indicated above, to draft initial responses to these questions, as well as eight additional subquestions that both the CMNR and BCNH felt needed to be addressed.

CONCLUSIONS AND RECOMMENDATIONS

• As recommended in earlier IOM reports (IOM, 1992a, 1995a), the importance of adequate nutrient intake (with sufficient energy to match output and to avoid weight loss) should be emphasized to soldiers as the primary means of maintaining lean tissue mass.

• Military researchers and physicians should pay careful attention to civilian research on the effects of treatment with anabolic hormones on recovery from burns and other injuries. Where appropriate, military-specific models should be developed.

• Current MRDAs for protein should be maintained. Provided that energy intake is adequate, no increase in MRDAs is necessary for pregnant or lactating women.

• Given adequate nutritional intake, soldiers should not use protein supplements for muscle building.

• Protein supplied in operational rations should be of high quality and digestibility.

• Energy intakes should be adequate, and a source of energy should be consumed within 2 h of an intense bout of endurance exercise, to replace depleted muscle glycogen.

• Single amino acid supplements should not be used to modify cognitive performance, due to potential toxicity and insufficient evidence of efficacy.

• The military should test the ability of supplemental glutamine and arginine to enhance the immune response and decrease rates of infection under field conditions and in seriously injured hospitalized patients.

• Given the high protein content of operational rations, adequate fluid intake should be emphasized, as recommended by the Fluid Doctrine (IOM, 1994).

* * * * *

The committee's responses to the questions, conclusions, and recommendations from this report are included in Appendix M.

References

AFEB (Armed Forces Epidemiological Board). 1996. Injuries in the military: a hidden epidemic. Report 29 HA 4844 97. Falls Church, Virg.: Armed Forces Epidemiologic Board.

AR (Army Regulation) 40-25. 1985. See U.S. Departments of the Army, the Navy, and the Air Force, 1985.

Cook, J.D., M. Carriaga, S.G. Kahn, W. Schalch, and B.S. Skikne. 1990. Gastric delivery system for iron supplementation. Lancet 335:1136–1139.

DHHS (Department of Health and Human Services). 1991. Healthy People 2000: National Health Promotion and Disease Prevention Objectives. DHHS Publication No. (PHS) 91-50213. Washington, D.C.: U.S. Government Printing Office.

Friedl, K.E., L.J. Marchitelli, D.E. Sherman, and R. Tulley. 1990. Nutritional assessment of cadets at the U.S. Military Academy: Part 1. Anthropometric & biochemical measures. Technical report T4-91. Natick, Mass.: U.S. Army Research Institute of Environmental Medicine.

IOM (Institute of Medicine). 1989. Plans for the Pennington Biomedical Research Center [letter report]. Committee on Military Nutrition Research, Food and Nutrition Board. June 26. Washington, D.C.

IOM. 1992a. Body Composition and Physical Performance, Applications for the Military Services, B.M. Marriott and J. Grumstrup-Scott, eds. Committee on Military Nutrition Research, Food and Nutrition Board. Washington, D.C.: National Academy Press.

IOM. 1992b. A Nutritional Assessment of U.S. Army Ranger Training Class 11/91. March 23. Washington, D.C.

IOM. 1992c. Research Progress Review of the Pennington Biomedical Research Center [letter report]. Committee on Military Nutrition Research, Food and Nutrition Board. May 15. Washington, D.C.

IOM. 1992d. Committee on Military Nutrition Research Review of Three Research Proposals from the Pennington Biomedical Research Center [letter report]. Committee on Military Nutrition Research, Food and Nutrition Board. December 10. Washington, D.C.

IOM. 1993a. Nutritional Needs in Hot Environments, Applications for Military Personnel in Field Environments, Bernadette M. Marriott, ed. Committee on Military Nutrition Research, Food and Nutrition Board. Washington, D.C.: National Academy Press.

IOM. 1993b. Review of the Results of Nutritional Intervention, U.S. Army Ranger Training Class 11/92 (Ranger II), B.M. Marriott, ed. Washington, D.C.: National Academy Press.

IOM. 1994a. Committee on Military Nutrition Research Activity Report, April 1, 1992–November 30, 1994, prepared by B.M. Marriott and P. Thomas. Committee on Military Nutrition Research, Food and Nutrition Board. Washington, D.C.: National Academy Press.

IOM. 1994b. Food Components to Enhance Performance, An Evaluation of Potential Performance-Enhancing Food Components for Operational Rations, B.M. Marriott, ed. Washington, D.C.: National Academy Press.

IOM. 1995a. Not Eating Enough, Overcoming Underconsumption of Military Operational Rations, Bernadette M. Marriott, ed. Committee on Military Nutrition Research, Food and Nutrition Board. Washington, D.C.: National Academy Press.

IOM. 1995b. Recommendations for Research on the Health of Military Women. Committee on Defense Women's Health Research, Food and Nutrition Board. Washington, D.C.: National Academy Press.

IOM. 1995c. A Review of the Revision of the Medical Services Nutrition Allowances, Standards, and Education (AR 40-25, 1985) [letter report]. Committee on Military Nutrition Research, Food and Nutrition Board. October 26. Washington, D.C.

IOM. 1995d. A Review of Issues Related to Iron Status in Women during U.S. Army Basic Combat Training [letter report]. Committee on Military Nutrition Research, Food and Nutrition Board. December 19. Washington, D.C.

IOM. 1996a. Nutritional Needs in Cold and in High-Altitude Environments, Applications for Military Personnel in Field Operations, Bernadette M. Marriott and Sydne J. Carlson, eds. Committee on Military Nutrition Research, Food and Nutrition Board. Washington, D.C.: National Academy Press.

IOM. 1996b. Pennington Biomedical Research Center September 1996 Site Visit [brief report]. Committee on Military Nutrition Research, Food and Nutrition Board. November 21. Washington, D.C.

IOM. 1997. Emerging Technologies for Nutrition Research: Potential for Assessing Military Performance Capability, Sydne J. Carlson-Newberry and Rebecca B. Costello, eds., Committee on Military Nutrition Research, Food and Nutrition Board. Washington, D.C.: National Academy Press.

IOM. 1998a. Assessing Readiness in Military Women: The Relationship of Body Composition, Nutrition, and Health. Subcommittee on Body Composition, Nutrition, and Health of Military Women. Washington, D.C.: National Academy Press.

IOM. 1998b. Reducing Stress Fractures in Physically Active Military Women [brief report]. Subcommittee on Body Composition, Nutrition, and Health of Military Women. Washington D.C.: National Academy Press.

IOM. 1999a. Antioxidants and Oxidative Stress in Military Personnel [letter report]. Committee on Military Nutrition Research, Food and Nutrition Board. February 12. Washington, D.C.

IOM. 1999b. Military Strategies for Sustainment of Nutrition and Immune Function in the Field. Committee on Military Nutrition Research, Food and Nutrition Board. Washington, D.C.: National Academy Press.

IOM. 1999c. The Role of Protein and Amino Acids in Sustaining and Enhancing Performance. Committee on Military Nutrition Research, Food and Nutrition Board. Washington, D.C.: National Academy Press.

Klicka, M.V., D.E. Sherman, N. King, K.E. Friedl, and E.W. Askew. 1993. Nutritional assessment of cadets at the U.S. Military Academy: Part 2. Assessment of Nutritional Intake. Technical report T94-1. Natick, Mass.: U.S. Army Research Institute of Environmental Medicine.

NRC (National Research Council). 1989a. Diet and Health: Implications for Reducing Chronic Disease Risk. Committee on Diet and Health, Food and Nutrition Board, Commission on Life Sciences. Washington, D.C.: National Academy Press.

NRC. 1989b. Recommended Dietary Allowances, 10th ed. Subcommittee on the Tenth Edition of the RDAs, Food and Nutrition Board, Commission on Life Sciences. Washington, D.C.: National Academy Press.

Shaffer, R.A. 1997. Physical training interventions to reduce stress fracture incidence in Navy and Marine Corps recruit training. Presentation at the workshop on Reducing Stress Fracture in Physically Active Young Servicemembers, December 10, Washington, D.C.

USDA (U.S. Department of Agriculture) and DHHS. 1995. Nutrition and Your Health: Dietary Guidelines for Americans, Fourth Edition. Home and Garden Bulletin No. 232. Washington, D.C.: U.S. Government Printing Office.

U.S. Departments of the Army, the Navy, and the Air Force. 1985. Army Regulation 40-25/Navy Command Medical Instruction 10110.1/Air Force Regulation 160-95. "Nutritional Allowances, Standards, and Education." May 15. Washington, D.C.

Westphal, K.A., L.J. Marchitelli, K.E. Friedl, and M.A. Sharp. 1995. Relationship between iron status and physical performance in female soldiers during U.S. Army Basic Combat Training [abstract]. Fed. Am. Soc. Exp. Biol. J. 9(3):A361.

Appendixes

A. Meetings of the Committee on Military Nutrition Research (including meetings of the Subcommittee on Body Composition, Nutrition, and Health of Military Women), December 1, 1994–May 31, 1999

B. Biographical Sketches of Members of the Committee on Military Nutrition Research, December 1, 1994–May 31, 1999

C. Conclusions and Recommendations from the Workshop Report *Not Eating Enough*, Submitted September 1995

D. Letter Report: *Review of the Revision of the Medical Services Nutrition Allowances, Standards*, and *Education* (AR 40-25, 1985), Submitted October 1995

E. Letter Report: *Review of Issues Related to Iron Status in Women During U.S. Army Basic Combat Training*, Submitted December 1995

F. Conclusions and Recommendations from the Workshop Report *Nutritional Needs in Cold and in High-Altitude Environments*, Submitted March 1996

G. Conclusions and Recommendations from the Brief Report *Pennington Biomedical Research Center September 1996 Site Visit*, Submitted November 1996

H. Conclusions and Recommendations from the Workshop Report *Emerging Technologies for Nutrition Research*, Submitted September 1997

I. Conclusions and Recommendations from the Workshop Report *Assessing Readiness in Military Women*, Submitted March 1998

J. Conclusions and Recommendations from the Brief Report: *Reducing Stress Fractures in Physically Active Military Women*, Submitted June 1998

K. Letter Report: *Antioxidants and Oxidative Stress in Military Personnel*, Submitted February, 1999

L. Conclusions and Recommendations from the Workshop Report: *Military Strategies for Sustainment of Nutrition and Immune Function in the Field*, Submitted May 1999

M. Conclusions and Recommendations from the Workshop Report: *The Role of Protein and Amino Acids in Sustaining and Enhancing Performance*, Submitted June 1999

Appendix A

Meetings of the Committee on Military Nutrition Research

December 1, 1994–May 31, 1999

Meetings of the Committee on Military Nutrition Research (including meetings of the Subcommittee on Body Composition, Nutrition, and Health of Military Women), December 1, 1994–May 31, 1999[*]

Dates	Topics	Location
January 26–27, 1995	CMNR Writing Session: *Not Eating Enough* *Nutritional Needs in Cold and in High-Altitude Environments*	Irvine, Calif.
May 22–24, 1995	CMNR Workshop and Committee Meeting: *Emerging Technologies for Nutrition Research*	Washington, D.C.
October 30, 1995	CMNR Workshop Planning Meeting (subcommittee): *Nutrition and Immune Function*	Irvine, Calif.
October 31, 1995	CMNR Planning Meeting (chair, sponsor, staff)	Washington, D.C.
November 1, 1995	BCNH Planning Meeting (chair, vice chair, sponsor, staff)	Washington, D.C.
November 13–14, 1995	CMNR Research Review Meeting: *A Review of Issues Related to Iron Status in Women During U.S. Army Basic Combat Training*	Washington, D.C.
March 21–22, 1996	CMNR Writing Session: *Emerging Technologies for Nutrition Research*	Washington, D.C.
April 12–13, 1996	BCNH Committee Meeting	Washington, D.C.
May 20–23, 1996	CMNR Workshop and Committee Meeting: *Nutrition and Immune Function*	Fort Detrick, Frederick, Md.

Continued

Meetings of the Committee on Military Nutrition Research (including meetings of the Subcommittee on Body Composition, Nutrition, and Health of Military Women), December 1, 1994–May 31, 1999[*] *Continued*

Dates	Topics	Location
September 9–11, 1996	BCNH Workshop and Committee Meeting: *Assessing Readiness in Military Women*	Irvine, Calif.
September 18–19, 1996	CMNR Research Review Meeting: *Pennington Biomedical Research Center September 1996 Site Visit*	Baton Rough, La.
	CMNR Writing Session: *Emerging Technologies for Nutrition Research Nutrition and Immune Function*	
January 29–30, 1997	CMNR Writing Session: *Nutrition and Immune Function*	Washington, D.C.
January 30–31, 1997	BCNH Writing Session: *Assessing Readiness in Military Women*	Washington, D.C.
March 13–14, 1997	CMNR-BCNH Workshop and Committee Meeting: *The Role of Protein and Amino Acids in Sustaining and Enhancing Performance*	Washington, D.C.
	CMNR Writing Session: *Nutrition and Immune Function*	
June 5–6, 1997	CMNR-BCNH Writing Session: *The Role of Protein and Amino Acids in Sustaining and Enhancing Performance*	Washington, D.C.

Meetings of the Committee on Military Nutrition Research (including meetings of the Subcommittee on Body Composition, Nutrition, and Health of Military Women), December 1, 1994–May 31, 1999* *Continued*

Dates	Topics	Location
June 18–19, 1997	BCNH Writing Session: *Assessing Readiness in Military Women*	Washington, D.C.
December 9–11, 1997	BCNH Workshop and Committee Meeting: *Reducing Stress Fracture in Physically Active Young Servicemembers*	Washington, D.C.
January 27, 1998	BCNH Writing Session: *Reducing Stress Fracture in Physically Active Young Servicewomen*	Palo Alto, Calif.
February 26, 1998	CMNR Planning Meeting (future chair, sponsor, staff)	Washington, D.C.
July 29–31, 1998	CMNR Workshop and Committee Meeting *Antioxidants and Oxidative Stress in Military Personnel*	Washington, D.C.
February 2–5, 1999	CMNR Workshop and Committee Meeting *Caffeine Formulations for Sustainment of Mental Task Performance in Military Operations*	Washington, D.C.

NOTE: CMNR, Committee on Military Nutrition Research; BCNH, Subcommittee on Body Composition, Nutrition, and Health of Military Women.

* Listed are all full committee meetings, workshops, planning meetings, subcommittee meetings, and larger workings sessions.

Biographical Sketches of Members of the Committee on Military Nutrition Research

December 1, 1994–May 31, 1999

Biographical Sketches of Members of the Committee on Military Nutrition Research[1]

JOHN E. VANDERVEEN (*Chair from July 1998*) is the retired Director of the Food and Drug Administration's (FDA) Office of Plant and Dairy Foods and Beverages in Washington, D.C. His previous position at the FDA was Director of the Division of Nutrition, at the Center for Food Safety and Applied Nutrition. He also served in various capacities at the U.S. Air Force (USAF) School of Aerospace Medicine at Brooks Air Force Base, Texas. He has received accolades for service from the FDA and the USAF. Dr. Vanderveen is a member of the American Society for Clinical Nutrition, American Institute of Nutrition, Aerospace Medical Association, American Dairy Science Association, Institute of Food Technologists, and American Chemical Society. In the past, he was the Treasurer of the American Society of Clinical Nutrition and a member of the Institute of Food Technology, National Academy of Sciences Advisory Committee. Dr. Vanderveen holds a B.S. in agriculture from Rutgers University, New Jersey and a Ph.D. in chemistry from the University of New Hampshire.

ROBERT O. NESHEIM (*Chair*) was Vice President of Research and Development and later Science and Technology for the Quaker Oats Company. He retired in 1983 and was Vice President of Science and Technology and President of the Advanced HealthCare Division of Avadyne, Inc. before his retirement in 1992. During World War II, he served as a captain in the U.S. Army. Dr. Nesheim has served on the Food and Nutrition Board (FNB), chairing the Committee on Food Consumption Patterns and serving as a member of several other committees. He also was active in the Biosciences Information Service (as Board Chairman), American Medical Association, American Institute of Nutrition, Institute of Food Technologists, and Food Reviews International

---

[1] Unless footnoted, affiliations listed correspond to initial committee membership period.

editorial board. Dr. Nesheim's academic services included Professor and Head of the Department of Animal Science at the University of Illinois, Urbana. He is a fellow of the American Institute of Nutrition and American Association for the Advancement of Science and a member of several professional organizations. Dr. Nesheim received a B.S. in agriculture, M.S. in animal science, and Ph.D. in nutrition and animal science from the University of Illinois.

LAWRENCE E. ARMSTRONG is an associate professor of exercise science at the University of Connecticut. He has joint appointments in the Department of Physiology and Neurobiology and the Department of Nutritional Sciences. Dr. Armstrong received his Ph.D. in human bioenergetics–exercise physiology from Ball State University. His research interests include thermoregulation, fluid-electrolyte balance, energy metabolism, exercise physiology, and the human heat illnesses. He previously served as a research physiologist at the U.S. Army Research Institute of Environmental Medicine. He is a fellow of the American College of Sports Medicine and a member of the Federation of American Societies for Experimental Biology and the Aerospace Medical Association.

RICHARD L. ATKINSON is Professor of Internal Medicine, Department of Nutrition Science at the University of Wisconsin-Madison. He was the Associate Chief of Staff for Research and Development at the Veterans Affairs Medical Center in Hampton, Virginia. Concurrently, Dr. Atkinson was Profes-sor of Internal Medicine and Chief of the Division of Clinical Nutrition at the Eastern Virginia Medical School in Norfolk, Virginia. He served 4 years in the military at Walter Reed Army Hospital in Washington, D.C. and the U.S. Army Hospital in Fort Campbell, Kentucky. Dr. Atkinson is an editorial board member for the *Journal of Nutrition*, a medical advisory board member for *Obesity Update*, and a contributing editor for *Nutrition Reviews*. He is a member of the American Association for the Advancement of Science, American Institute of Nutrition, and Endocrine Society; he is a fellow of the American College of Nutrition and American College of Physicians. Dr. Atkinson holds a B.A. from the Virginia Military Institute in Lexington and M.D. from the Medical College of Virginia in Richmond, where he served his internship. He then completed his residency at Harbor General Hospital in Torrance, California.

WILLIAM R. BEISEL is Adjunct Professor in the Department of Molecular Microbiology and Immunology at The Johns Hopkins University School of Hygiene and Public Health. He held several positions at the U.S. Army Medical Research Institute of Infectious Diseases at Fort Detrick, Maryland, including in turn, Chief of the Physical Sciences Division, Scientific Advisor, and Deputy for Science. He then became Special Assistant for Biotechnology to the Surgeon General. After serving in the U.S. military during the Korean War, Dr. Beisel was the Chief of Medicine at the U.S. Army Hospital in Fort Leonard Wood,

Missouri, before becoming the Chief of the Department of Metabolism at the Walter Reed Army Hospital. He was awarded a Commendation Ribbon, Bronze Star for the Korean War, Hoff Gold Medal at the Walter Reed Army Institute of Research, B. L. Cohen Award of the American Society for Microbiology, the Robert Herman Award from the American Association for Clinical Nutrition, and Department of Army Decoration for Exceptional Civilian Service. He was named a diplomat of the American Board of Internal Medicine and a fellow of the American College of Physicians. In addition to his many professional memberships, Dr. Beisel is a *Clinical Nutrition* contributing editor and *Journal of Nutritional Immunology* associate editor. He received his A.B. from Muhlenberg College in Allentown, Pennsylvania, and M.D. from the Indiana University School of Medicine.

GAIL E. BUTTERFIELD is Director of Nutrition Research, Palo Alto Veterans Affairs Health Care System in California. Concurrently, she is Lecturer in the Department of Medicine, Stanford University Medical School; Visiting Assistant Professor in the Program of Human Biology, Stanford University; and Director of Nutrition in the Program in Sports Medicine, Stanford University Medical School. Her previous academic appointments were at the University of California, Berkeley. Dr. Butterfield belongs to the American Institute of Nutrition, American Society for Clinical Nutrition, American Dietetic Association, and American Physiological Society. As a fellow of the American College of Sports Medicine, she serves as Chair of the Pronouncements Committee and was recently elected Vice President; she also was President and Executive Director of the Southwest Chapter of that organization. She is a member of the Respiratory and Applied Physiology Study Section of the NIH and is on the editorial boards of the following journals: *Medicine and Science in Sports and Exercise, Health and Fitness Journal of ACSM, Canadian Journal of Clinical Sports Medicine,* and *International Journal of Sports Nutrition.* Dr. Butterfield earned her A.B. in biological sciences, M.A. in anatomy, and M.S. and Ph.D. in nutrition from the University of California, Berkeley, and she is a registered dietitian. Her current research interests include nutrition in exercise, effect of growth factors on protein metabolism in the elderly, and metabolic fuel use in women exposed to high altitude.

WANDA L. CHENOWETH is Professor in the Department of Food Science and Human Nutrition at Michigan State University. Previously, she held positions as Teaching Associate at the University of Iowa and University of California, Berkeley. Other work experience includes positions as Research Dietitian and Head Clinical Dietitian at University of Iowa Hospitals and as Research Dietitian at Mayo Clinic. She is a member of the American Society for Nutritional Sciences, American Dietetic Association, and Institute of Food Technology. She serves as a reviewer for several journals, including *Journal of* *the American Dietetic Association, American Journal of Clinical Nutrition, Journal of Nutrition,* and is a member of the associate editorial board of *Plant Foods for Human Nutrition.* She has served on a technical review committee for the Diet, Nutrition, and Cancer Program of the National Cancer Institute and as a Site Evaluator, Commission on Evaluation of Dietetic Education of the American Dietetic Association. Her research interests are in the area of mineral bioavailability and clinical nutrition. Dr. Chenoweth completed a B.S. in dietetics from the University of Iowa, dietetic internship and M.S. in nutrition at the University of Iowa, and Ph.D. in nutrition at the University of California, Berkeley.

JOHN D. FERNSTROM is Professor of Psychiatry, Pharmacology, and Behavioral Neuroscience at the University of Pittsburgh School of Medicine and Director, Basic Neuroendocrinology Program at the Western Psychiatric Institute and Clinic. He received his B.S. in biology and his Ph.D. in nutritional biochemistry from the Massachusetts Institute of Technology (M.I.T.). He was a Postdoctoral Fellow in Neuroendocrinology at the Roche Institute for Molecular Biology in Nutley, New Jersey. Before coming to the University of Pittsburgh, Dr. Fernstrom was an Assistant and then Associate Professor in the Department of Nutrition and Food Science at M.I.T. He has served on numerous governmental advisory committees. He presently is a member of the National Advisory Council of the Monell Chemical Senses Center, Chair of the Neurosciences Section of the American Society for Nutritional Sciences (ASNS), and a member of the ASNS Council. He is a member of numerous professional societies, including the American Institute of Nutrition, American Society for Clinical Nutrition, American Physiological Society, American Society for Pharmacology and Experimental Therapeutics, American Society for Neurochemistry, Society for Neuroscience, and Endocrine Society. Among other awards, Dr. Fernstrom received the Mead-Johnson Award of the American Institute of Nutrition, a Research Scientist Award from the National Institute of Mental Health, a Wellcome Visiting Professorship in the Basic Medical Sciences, and an Alfred P. Sloan Fellowship in Neurochemistry. His current major research interest concerns the influence of the diet and drugs on the synthesis of neurotransmitters in the central and peripheral nervous systems.

JOËL A. GRINKER is Professor of Pediatrics and Communicable Diseases at the School of Public Health, University of Michigan-Ann Arbor. She is a member of the university's Center for Human Growth and Development and served as Director of the Program in Human Nutrition. She was Visiting Scientist at the USDA Human Nutrition Research Center on Aging at Tufts University in Boston and Visiting Associate Professor at the Lavaratoire de Neurophysiologie Sensorielle et Comportementale, College de France, Paris. Currently, she is a reviewer for the National Cancer Institute, National Institutes of Health, and National Science Foundation and for several professional journals. She serves on the editorial boards for *Appetite, Journal of Eating Disorders*, and *Psychosomatic Medicine*. She is a fellow of the American Psychological Association, American Association for the Advancement of Science, and New York Academy of Sciences and is a member of several professional societies. Dr. Grinker holds a B.A. in Experimental Social Psychology from New York University. At Rockefeller University, she was a Russell Sage Post-doctoral Fellow in the Laboratory of Human Behavior and Metabolism of Dr. Jules Hirsch and then Assistant and Associate Professor.

G. RICHARD JANSEN is Professor Emeritus in the Department of Food Science and Human Nutrition at Colorado State University, where he was Head of the department from 1969 to 1990. He was a Research Fellow at the Merck Institute for Therapeutic Research and Senior Research Biochemist in the Electrochemical Department at E. I. DuPont de Nemours. Prior to his stint in private industry, he served in the U.S. Air Force. Dr. Jansen is a past member of the U.S. Department of Agriculture (USDA) Human Nutrition Board of Scientific Counselors and the *Journal of Nutrition, Nutrition Reports International*, and *Plant Foods for Human Nutrition* editorial boards. His research interests deal with protein energy relationships during lactation and new foods for developing countries based on low-cost extrusion cooking. He received the Babcock-Hart Award of the Institute of Food Technologists and a Certificate of Merit from the USDA's Office of International Cooperation and Development for his work on low-cost extrusion cooking, and he is an IFT Fellow. He is a member of the American Society for Nutritional Sciences, Institute of Food Technologists, and American Society for Biochemistry and Molecular Biology among others. Dr. Jansen holds a B.A. in chemistry and Ph.D. in biochemistry from Cornell University in Ithaca, New York.

ROBIN B. KANAREK is Professor of Psychology and of Nutrition at Tufts University in Medford, Massachusetts, where she also is the Chair of Psychology. Her prior experience includes Research Fellow, Division of Endocrinology, UCLA School of Medicine and Research Fellow in Nutrition at Harvard University. In addition to reviewing for several journals, including *Science, Brain Research Bulletin, Journal of Nutrition, American Journal of Clinical Nutrition*, and *Annals of Internal Medicine*, she is an editorial board member of *Physiology and Behavior* and the *Tufts Diet and Nutrition Newsletter* and is a past editor-in-chief of *Nutrition and Behavior*. Dr. Kanarek has served on ad hoc review committees for the National Science Foundation, NIH, and USDA Nutrition Research, as well as the Member Program Committee of the Eastern Psychological Association. She is a Fellow of the American College of Nutrition, and her other professional memberships include the American Institute of Nutrition, New York Academy of Sciences, Society for the Study of

Ingestive Behavior, and Society for Neurosciences. Dr. Kanarek received a B.A. in biology from Antioch College in Yellow Springs, Ohio and M.S. and Ph.D. in psychology from Rutgers University in New Brunswick, New Jersey.

ORVILLE A. LEVANDER is Research Leader for USDA Nutrient Requirements and Functions Laboratory in Beltsville, Maryland. He was Research Chemist at the USDA's Human Nutrition Research Center, Resident Fellow in Biochemistry at Columbia University's College of Physicians and Surgeons, and Research Associate at Harvard University's School of Public Health. Dr. Levander served on the Food and Nutrition Board's Committee on the Dietary Allowances. He also served on panels of the National Research Council's Committee on Animal Nutrition and Committee on the Biological Effects of Environmental Pollutants. He was a member of the U.S. National Committee for the International Union of Nutrition Sciences and temporary advisor to the World Health Organization's Environmental Health Criteria Document on Selenium. Dr. Levander was awarded the Osborne and Mendel Award of the American Institute of Nutrition. His society memberships include the American Institute of Nutrition, American Chemical Society, and American Society for Clinical Nutrition. Dr. Levander received his B.A. from Cornell University and his M.S. and Ph.D. in biochemistry from the University of Wisconsin-Madison.

GILBERT A. LEVEILLE recently retired as Vice President for Research and Technical Services at the Nabisco Foods Group in East Hanover, New Jersey. His other industry experience was as the Director of Nutrition and Health Science for the General Foods Corporation. He was Chair and Professor of Food Science and Human Nutrition at Michigan State University, Professor of Nutritional Biochemistry at the University of Illinois-Urbana, and a Biochemist at the U.S. Army Medical Research and Nutrition Laboratory in Colorado. Dr. Leveille was a member of the Committee on International Nutrition, a joint Food and Nutrition Board-Board on International Health project. He won a research award from the Poultry Science Association, the Mead Johnson Research Award from the American Institute of Nutrition, the Distinguished Faculty Award from Michigan State University, and the Carl R. Fellers Award from the Institute of Food Technologists. He is a member of the American Association for the Advancement of Science, American Institute of Nutrition (Past President), American Society for Clinical Nutrition, American Chemical Society, Institute of Food Technologists (Past President), and Sigma Xi. Dr. Leveille received his B.V.A. from the University of Massachusetts and M.S. and Ph.D. in nutrition and biochemistry from Rutgers University, New Jersey.

ESTHER STERNBERG is chief of the Section on Neuroendocrine Immunology and Behavior and associate branch chief of the Clinical Neuroendocrinology Branch of the National Institutes of Mental Health

Intramural Research Program at the National Institute of Health (NIH). Dr. Sternberg received her M.D. degree and trained in rheumatology at McGill University, Montreal, Canada. She did postdoctoral training at Washington University, Barnes Hospital, St. Louis, Missouri, in the Division of Allergy and Immunology. She was subsequently a Howard Hughes associate and instructor in medicine at Washington University and Barnes Hospital before joining NIH. Dr. Sternberg is internationally recognized for her ground-breaking discoveries in the area of central nervous system–immune system interactions. She has received the Arthritis Foundation William R. Felts Award for Excellence in Rheumatology Research Publications, has been awarded the Public Health Service Superior Service Award, and has been elected to the American Society for Clinical Investigation in recognition of this work. Dr. Sternberg is also internationally recognized as a foremost authority on the l-tryptophan eosinophilia–myalgia syndrome (L-TRP-EMS). She was the first to describe this syndrome in relation to a similar drug l-5-hydroxytryptophan, and published this landmark article in the *New England Journal of Medicine* in 1980.

DOUGLAS W. WILMORE, the Frank Sawyer Professor of Surgery at Harvard Medical School, is a Senior Staff Scientist and Surgeon at Brigham and Women's Hospital, Boston, Massachusetts. Concurrently, he is also a consultant for the Dana-Farber Cancer Center, Children's Hospital Medical Center, the BI-Deaconess Hospital, Wrentham State School, and Youville Hospital and Rehabilitation Center. Dr. Wilmore's main interests are related to metabolic and nutritional means to support critically ill patients and enhance recovery. His basic research has been applied to patients with thermal and accidental injury, patients with infectious complications, and those with multiple organ failure. He worked with the team that developed the current method of intravenous nutrition used for patients throughout the world. This technique has been improved in Dr. Wilmore's laboratory, and new amino acid solutions have been developed utilizing the amino acid glutamine, and anabolic factors such as growth hormone have been incorporated in this new feeding program with dramatic therapeutic results. Dr. Wilmore serves on the advisory board of the Tufts Pediatric Trauma Center, international editorial committee of the *Chinese Nutritional Sciences Journal of the Chinese Academy of Medical Sciences*, and editorial boards of *Annals of Surgery* and *Journal of the American College of Surgeons*. He is senior editor of Scientific American Surgery, the surgical text published by the American College of Surgeons that serves as the basis for care of general surgical patients. He also has published over 300 scientific papers and 4 books. Among his professional memberships, Dr. Wilmore includes the American College of Surgeons, American Surgical Association, American Medical Association, Society of University Surgeons, and American Society for Parenteral and Enteral Nutrition. He holds a B.A. and honorary Ph.D. from

Washburn University of Topeka, M.D. from the University of Kansas School of Medicine in Kansas City, and honorary M.S. from Harvard University.

JOHANNA T. DWYER (*FNB Liaison*) is the Director of the Frances Stern Nutrition Center at New England Medical Center and Professor in the Departments of Medicine and of Community Health at the Tufts Medical School and School of Nutrition Science and Policy in Boston. She is also Senior Scientist at the Jean Mayer/USDA Human Nutrition Research Center on Aging at Tufts. Dr. Dwyer is the author or coauthor of more than 120 research articles and 200 review articles published in scientific journals. Her work centers on life-cycle related concerns such as the prevention of diet-related disease in children and adolescents and maximization of quality of life and health in the elderly. She also has a longstanding interest in vegetarian and other alternative lifestyles.

Dr. Dwyer is a past President of the American Institute of Nutrition, past Secretary of the American Society for Clinical Nutrition, and past President and current Fellow of the Society for Nutrition Education. She served on the Program Development Board of the American Public Health Association from 1989 to 1992 and is a member of the Food and Nutrition Board, the Technical Advisory Committee of the Nutrition Screening Initiative, and the Board of Directors of the American Institute of Wine and Food. As a Robert Wood Johnson Health Policy Fellow (1980–1981), she served on the personal staffs of Senator Richard Lugar (R-Indiana) and Senator Barbara Mikulski (D-Maryland). She was recently elected to the Institute of Medicine.

Dr. Dwyer has received numerous honors and awards for her work in the field of nutrition, including the 1996 W. O. Atwater Award of the USDA and J. Harvey Wiley Award from the Society for Nutrition Education. She gave the Lenna Frances Cooper Lecture at the annual meeting of the American Dietetic Association in 1990. Dr. Dwyer is currently editor of *Nutrition Today*, on the editorial board for *Family Economics* and *Nutrition Review* and advisory board for *Clinics in Applied Nutrition*, and is a contributing editor for *Nutrition Reviews*, as well as a reviewer for the *Journal of the American Dietetic Association*, *American Journal of Clinical Nutrition*, and *American Journal of Public Health*. She received her D.Sc. and M.Sc. from the Harvard School of Public Health, an M.S. from the University of Wisconsin, and completed her undergraduate degree with distinction from Cornell University.

REBECCA B. COSTELLO (*FNB Staff, Project Director from July 15, 1996 through May 23, 1998*) is Project Director for the Committee on Military Nutrition Research (CMNR) and Subcommittee on Body Composition, Nutrition, and Health of Military Women (BCNH). Prior to joining the FNB staff, she served as Research Associate and Program Director for the Risk Factor Reduction Center, a referral center for the detection, modification, and prevention of cardiovascular disease through dietary and/or drug interventions at the Washington Adventist Hospital in Takoma Park, Maryland. She received her B.S. and M.S. in biology from the American University, Washington, D.C., and a Ph.D. in clinical nutrition from the University of Maryland at College Park. She has active membership in the American Institute of Nutrition, American College of Nutrition, American Dietetic Association, and American Heart Association Council on Epidemiology. Dr. Costello's areas of research interest include mineral nutrition, dietary intake methodology, and chronic disease epidemiology.

SYDNE J. CARLSON-NEWBERRY (*FNB Staff, Program Officer*) is Program Officer for the CMNR and BCNH. Prior to joining the FNB staff, she served as Project Director for the Women's Health Project and Adjunct Assistant Professor in the Department of Family Medicine, Wright State University School of Medicine; as a behavioral health educator for a hospital-based weight management program in Dayton, Ohio; and as a research associate at The Ohio State University Biotechnology Center. She received her B.A. from Brandeis University and her Ph.D. in nutritional biochemistry and metabolism from M.I.T. and completed a NIH postdoctoral fellowship in the Departments of Biochemistry and Molecular Genetics at Ohio State. Dr. Carlson-Newberry's areas of research interest include eating disorders and diabetes management.

BERNADETTE M. MARRIOTT (*FNB Staff, Project Director through November 22, 1995*) is former Director of the Office of Dietary Supplements Research at NIH and was Project Director for the CMNR and Deputy Director of the FNB. She has a Ph.D. in psychology from the University of Aberdeen, Scotland, and B.Sc. in biochemistry/immunology and postdoctoral laboratory training in comparative medicine and trace mineral nutrition. She serves on the Scientific Advisory board for the Diagon Corporation and the American Health Foundation. She serves as scientific reviewer for the NIH, National Science Foundation, and National Geographic. Prior to joining the Institute of Medicine staff, she held university and medical school faculty positions at the Johns Hopkins University, University of Puerto Rico School of Medicine, and Goucher College. Her areas of research interest include bioenergetic modeling, trace mineral nutrition, and ingestive behavior in human and nonhuman primates.

MARY I. POOS (*FNB Staff, Project Director, since May 23, 1998*) is project director for the Committee on Military Nutrition Research (CMNR). She joined the Food and Nutrition Board of the Institute of Medicine in November 1997. She has been a project director for the National Academy of Sciences since 1990. Prior to officially joining the FNB staff, she served as a project director for the National Research Council's Board on Agriculture for more than seven years, two of which were spent on loan to the FNB. Her work with the FNB includes senior staff officer for the IOM report *The Program of Research for Military Nursing* and study director for the reports *A Review of the Department of Defense's Program for Breast Cancer Research* and *Vitamin C Fortification of Food Aid Commodities*. Currently, she also serves as study director to the Subcommittee on Interpretation and Uses of Dietary Reference Intakes. While working with the Board on Agriculture, Dr. Poos was responsible for the Committee on Animal Nutrition and directed the production of seven reports in the *Nutrient Requirements of Domestic Animals* series, including a letter report to the commissioner of FDA concerning the importance of selenium in animal nutrition. Prior to joining the National Academy of Sciences she was consultant/owner of Nutrition Consulting Services of Greenfield, Massachusetts; assistant professor in the Department of Veterinary and Animal Sciences at the University of Massachusetts, Amherst; and adjunct assistant professor in the Department of Animal Sciences, University of Vermont. She received her B.S. in biology from Virginia Polytechnic Institute and State University, and a Ph.D. in animal sciences (nutrition/biochemistry) from the University of Kentucky; she completed a postdoctoral fellowship in the Department of Animal Sciences Area of Excellence Program at the University of Nebraska. Dr. Poos's areas of research interest include protein and nitrogen metabolism and nutrition–reproduction interactions.

Appendix C

Conclusions and Recommendations from the Workshop Report Not Eating Enough

Submitted September 1995

Committee Responses to Questions, Conclusions, and Recommendations

As stated in Chapter 1, the Committee on Military Nutrition Research (CMNR) was asked to address five specific questions dealing with strategies to overcome underconsumption of military operational rations. The committee's responses to these questions appear below. These answers are further elaborated in the recommendations that follow. The conclusions and areas for research developed by the CMNR are also included.

ANSWERS TO THE QUESTIONS POSED TO THE COMMITTEE

1. Why do soldiers underconsume (not meet energy expenditure needs) in field operations?

Ration factors, including palatability, variety, and temperature of the foods, are major contributors to general acceptance. Heavy activity or environmental extremes may increase energy requirements without compensating ration intake. Hypohydration may lead to temporary anorexia and a worsening cycle of lowered water and food intake. However, environmental or logistic components that are often under the influence or control of the command are also extremely important. These factors include such situational elements as designation of eating locations, meal schedules, social setting (alone or with others), and provision of rations at appropriate temperatures. The committee believes that multiple logistic, situational, and sensory factors contribute to decreased consumption. Military operational rations are by design all inclusive and do not allow substitution or choice. Failure to provide adequate time, instruction, and encouragement to eat and drink can materially influence consumption. The attitude of the local commander is critical in ensuring that soldiers are aware that daily adequate nutrition is important so as not to degrade performance over a period of time. It would be an important future research step to provide a priority order for the impact of these multiple factors on soldier food intake in the field.

2. What factors influence underconsumption in field operations? Identify the relative importance of rations, environment, the eating situation, and the individual.

A number of factors influence the quantity of operational rations consumed. Generally under field conditions, an underconsumption of rations is observed, which leads to weight loss. Numerous factors including the environment, the specific eating situation, the ration itself, and the individual can affect the amount of rations that will be consumed. Any one of these can be the most important factor depending on the situation. Further review of the relevant military data on eating situations that provides an integrated overview of the ordering of environment, the rations, and the individual factors with situational change would be beneficial. The following are reasonable conclusions/opinions based on available evidence:

Environment: Field environments are generally harsh, frequently require increased energy expenditure, and are not conducive to the enjoyment of eating. Proximity to danger, temperature extremes, unappetizing local conditions, and lack of protection from the elements are all conditions that are encountered in a military scenario and can contribute to an impairment of appetite and underconsumption.

Eating Situation: The opportunity for social interaction, information exchange, and appropriateness of meal to the time of day, are all elements of the eating situation that can contribute to food intake.

Rations: Acceptability of rations to the soldier includes temperature, sensory properties (taste, smell, texture, color, and temperature), packaging, individual food preferences, ease of use, nutritional content, stability of product, appropriateness to time of day, delivery, presentation, availability, variety, and duration of reliance on operational rations as a major source of available food.

Individual: The individual soldier's attitude toward military feeding systems is an important determinant of ration consumption. The commander's attitude regarding the feeding system and his or her knowledge of nutrition may influence the soldier's eating behavior. Activities of the individual soldier, such as consuming adequate fluids, drinking when eating, taking advantage of opportunities to heat appropriate ration components, and snacking on certain ration items when opportunities permit, will enhance energy consumption and nutrient intake.

3. At what level of underconsumption is there a negative impact on physical or cognitive performance?

Underconsumption of fluid or working in hot environmental conditions, either as a result of protective clothing or atmospheric conditions, may result in weight losses of 3 to 5 percent in less than 48 hours and can significantly reduce physical and cognitive performance. Therefore maintaining adequate hydration is critical to maintaining performance.

Existing historical and experimental data indicate that decrements in physical performance begin in well-hydrated individuals when 10 percent or more of initial weight has been lost. Other studies suggest that losses as great as 15 percent do not result in decrements in physical performance, if lean body mass is preserved and if the weight loss is primarily from body fat stores. Similarly, decrements in cognitive performance appear to begin to occur when weight losses reach 10 percent of baseline. It is likely that greater losses of body fat will not affect cognitive performance, if lean body mass is preserved. There is only limited, well-controlled research available, however, that addresses this issue. With both physical and cognitive performance, the key factors that must be considered are the initial body composition of the individual and the rate of weight loss. Active military personnel who meet the height and weight standards for their age are relatively lean with some soldiers having as little as 10 percent body fat. Rapid weight loss (in excess of 2 lb/wk) in such lean individuals indicates significant underconsumption with regard to energy expenditure and can be expected to lead to decrements in performance.

Intakes of protein in excess of normal intake may help preserve muscle mass in circumstances of inadequate energy intake but will not totally prevent its loss. Adequate carbohydrate intake, particularly during or following periods of heavy physical activity, will aid in maintaining or restoring muscle glycogen and maintaining performance.

4. Given the environment of military operations, what steps are suggested to enhance ration consumption? To overcome deficits in food intake? To overcome any degradation in physical or cognitive performance?

Adequate fluid intake to prevent dehydration is the first step to prevent or overcome deficits in performance since the consequences of dehydration are most immediate. In addition, as noted in the foregoing discussion, there are many other factors that affect ration consumption in the environment of military operations. They include, but are not limited to, the nature of the rations; the eating situation in which such rations must be consumed; the environmental conditions that influence how, when, and under what physical conditions (i.e., temperature) the rations will be consumed; and the motivation provided the soldier to consume the food. To overcome possible effects of underconsumption on physical and cognitive performance, efforts should continue to increase the overall consumption of rations by military personnel in the field through a variety of approaches, which include establishing a *field feeding doctrine* at all levels within the command structure down to the individual soldier. Such a *field feeding doctrine* would include definitions of adequate food intake for soldiers in military operations and the potential consequences to performance and health of not eating enough. Steps to assure that soldiers have adequate intake should also be outlined in the food doctrine.

Military operational rations must be designed so as to protect body weight, especially lean body mass, by ensuring an adequate intake of energy, carbohydrate, protein, vitamins, and minerals. In considering the nature of the ration, continued effort to improve flavor, texture, and other organoleptic qualities should be pursued. The CMNR believes that current rations are of very high quality given what they are designed to do. Efforts to provide enhancements that will alter the flavor of entree items through the use of seasonings and other condiments should receive continued research and development. Use of newer processing technology should also be integrated into current rations to preserve greater texture of thermostabilized foods, which are packaged in flexible containers. Finally, research should be continued to provide greater stabilization of fat within other food components to reduce the appearance and mouth feel of greasiness in high-fat foods.

Although the extent to which the eating situation can be changed may be limited, making specific time available for eating is important and perhaps critical. Ideally soldiers should be able to eat in groups, and the opportunity to interact and share experiences should be provided when the tactical situation permits.

Steps should also be taken to cope with environmental factors that detract from food acceptance. For example, continued development of equipment for heating and preparing foods that can be used in remote locations and extreme environments, and improvement in individual equipment for preparing meals, should be undertaken. With indication from existing military and commercial research that "nibbling" can play an important role in overall energy intake, consideration should be given to the development of additional ration components that can be readily stored in pockets and consumed at a later time, especially high calorie and nutrient rich beverages of high acceptability.

Finally, steps should be taken to motivate soldiers to consume sufficient quantities of food to more nearly match their energy expenditures and maintain optimal performance. This motivation would be fostered by education and by encouragement through command leadership. The soldier should be provided information about the physiological and functional consequences of underconsumption of rations. Commanders should emphasize the quality of the food system and thereby create a positive image for the ration. The entire command structure should be involved in this effort. Special training on the importance of nutrition in maintaining physical and cognitive performance and morale should be provided to all command personnel. Platoon sergeants should be capable of informing their soldiers about their needs for adequate energy and water intake. The ultimate goal should be that ration consumption should be given equal priority to other training needs of the soldier.

The image of the ration both for the civilian and the soldier should also be improved. Current new endeavors incorporating humor with a nutrition and performance message into films appear to be a positive step if the impact of these films is carefully measured and the education message is retained. Changing the labeling of the individual food items will also be helpful. More information about the nutrient content and on alternative means of preparation of the entree should be included. Although outer packaging may have to comply with camouflage requirements, more colorful labeling of internal packaging would provide greater product appeal and relief from monotony.

5. What further research needs to be done in these areas?

This question will be addressed in the last section of this chapter, Areas for Future Research.

CONCLUSIONS

The Underconsumption Problem

Studies of field training exercises typically report underconsumption of military operational rations. Underconsumption in this context has been defined as an energy intake insufficient to meet the needs of the energy expenditure. The consequence is weight loss, with the amount of the weight loss being proportional to the underconsumption of energy from the ration. In six studies where the doubly labeled water method was used to measure energy expenditure, the Meal, Ready-to-Eat (MRE) intakes were compared with other ration combinations during field training exercises lasting from 10 to 30 days. An average underconsumption of approximately 1,552 kcal/d (range 520–2,199 kcal/d) relative to measured energy expenditure was demonstrated. All but one of these studies were conducted under conditions known to markedly increase energy requirements (BMR elevated 20–40 percent) and have shown energy consumption ranging from 52 to 85 percent of energy expenditure. In a series of short-term studies with research modifications of the MRE ration, there has been improved energy intake with each MRE version (for example, MRE IV and MRE improved, MRE VIII and supplement, etc.). However, it is not known if this increase is sustained over longer-term use in the field or represents a novelty effect. Both consumer and military research has indicated that some ration components such as bread, high-starch vegetables, and certain beverages can be expected to retain their high acceptance.

In contrast, limited studies using A Rations or mixed rations in field settings have shown energy intakes approximating energy expenditure (cf., Rose and Carlson, 1986). Therefore, it appears that under certain conditions, consumption of rations in the field can equal energy expenditure. It should be recognized that a comparison of field exercises that provide A Rations, which consist of hot and/or fresh foods, with those that supply only MREs represent measurement of ration acceptance confounded with other variables. Factors other than ration quality or food acceptance including food temperature and variety, as well as situational factors and logistics, can have a major impact on consumption of military operational rations.

Potential Effects of Underconsumption on Performance

The significance of underconsumption, with its consequent loss in body weight, is its impact on physical and cognitive performance. The MRE studies show that while daily energy deficits of 1,000 to 1,500 kcal/d occurred, protein and other major nutrient intakes remained at basically adequate levels. Thus, during periods of from 30 to 42 days, deficiencies of nutrients other than energy are unlikely when consuming the MRE ration.

The rate of weight loss must be considered in addressing the potential impacts of underconsumption on performance. In physically fit and healthy troops rapid weight loss of 3 to 5 percent in less than 48 hours is primarily due to dehydration and can impact on physical and cognitive performance. Weight loss in excess of 5 percent in this time frame will most likely be associated with decreased performance and can lead to negative effects on health.

In initially well-nourished and properly hydrated troops, weight losses not associated with trauma or disease reflect the deficit in energy intake relative to expenditure. Therefore rapid weight loss (in excess of 2 lb/wk) indicate significant underconsumption of energy (1,000 or more kcal/d). A loss of 10 percent of body weight in a soldier of initial weight of 160 lb in just 4 weeks reflects a kcal deficit in the range of 2,000 kcal/d. If weight losses are modest in the range of 1 lb/wk the loss will primarily be from body fat. More rapid losses, particularly in lean individuals, will reflect a greater loss of lean body mass in addition to body fat. Weight losses primarily from body fat are not likely to reduce performance; however, as weight losses increase and an increasing percent of the loss is from muscle tissue, measured decreases in performance will occur as shown in the studies reported by Friedl (see Chapter 14 in this volume). Soldiers with lower body fat will lose more lean muscle mass from the beginning than those with higher fat reserves (Vanderveen et al., 1977). Given the individual variation in body composition of physically fit soldiers, it is not possible to specifically relate potential performance deficit to a specific percent loss of body weight, particularly in a period of 4 to 6 weeks. The problem is further complicated by the possibility of an individual, who may have lost 5 to 10 percent of body weight in a deployment, being redeployed before sufficient time to regain the lost weight. The individual will face a further weight loss with lower fat reserves and consequently lose lean body mass with even a relatively small loss of body weight.

Therefore it seems prudent to minimize body weight losses when possible during operations to maintain a high degree of fitness and performance. This may be particularly important in the current downsizing of the forces as units may be frequently deployed as the need arises in various parts of the world.

Very limited data are available on the impact of weight losses on cognitive performance. Closely related are potential mood or morale changes that may adversely affect cognitive performance. Therefore, careful attention to the weight changes in a unit during extended operational deployment is important to assure that operational capability is maintained.

Strategies to Overcome Underconsumption

Underconsumption of military operational rations is undoubtedly a multifaceted problem:

• Ration factors, such as ration image, palatability of individual components, nutrient density, variety, meal and meal item appropriateness for the time of day, and fluid intake, contribute to the general level of acceptance.

• Situational factors, such as eating location, social setting, and allowing sufficient time to eat and drink during deployment and in the field, as well as appropriate meal scheduling with consideration of changes in circadian rhythms, are likely to be important.

• Environmental factors, such as protection from heat or cold, ability to heat entree components or consume fluid products at appropriate temperatures, and the accessibility of fluids, influence food intake.

• Emotional state, such as feelings of security from enemy action, can affect appetite and ingestive behavior.

• Leadership issues, such as influence of the unit commander on soldier attitudes toward ration consumption, can be critical. Positive attitudes expressed by officers and noncommissioned officers can influence intake. Commanders may be influenced by effects of ration intake on morale and/or on physical and cognitive performance over a period of time. A subset of the leadership issue is individual soldier attitude.

An important step in developing strategies to overcome underconsumption of military operational rations is to analyze critically the available data. Such analysis should help identify the potential contribution of the factors outlined above to the underconsumption issue. This analysis will serve two important purposes. *First*, those factors relating to ration, situation, environment, and leadership that appear to bear the greatest impact within each category could be identified and quantified to the extent possible. Then a *field feeding doctrine* could be developed in which each of these major factors is quantified, enabling field commanders to make informed choices relative to the situations in the military operation.

Significant efforts on the part of the U.S. Army Natick Research, Development and Engineering Center (NRDEC) to improve the acceptability of rations, particularly the MRE, have resulted in a demonstrated improvement in intake in experimental field settings. The MRE has great flexibility in its pattern of use; for example, it can be eaten by the individual soldier while on the move, in isolation, and without heating. This scenario will likely result in the least favorable consumption of the ration. However, if the combat situation permits, combat units (squad, platoon, and companies) could be permitted to come together at a scheduled time to consume their MREs in a more favorable social and environmental situation. Given this context, MRE consumption is likely to be higher than when eaten in isolation, and the troops will remain in a potentially better nutritional condition for forthcoming operations.

Second, constructing a ration consumption model in which the incremental effects of the various factors that may influence intake relative to need are identified and quantified would help to delineate the state of current scientific knowledge. Gaps that exist (presumably with an indication of the relative importance of each to facilitate setting research priorities) could be identified and a research agenda developed. Information gleaned from this model would be an important step in developing a *field feeding doctrine.*

The development of the new concept in the Army Field Feeding System as outlined by Peter Motrynczuk in Chapter 4 would reduce the long-term dependence on the MRE and, at least in theory, overcome some of the concerns over the weight losses due to underconsumption observed in the field studies. The highly engineered MRE system has functioned very well in fulfilling the original concept of a highly portable, nutritionally adequate ration for use in the initial stages of a military operation. The decision by senior Army leadership to implement this new field feeding system will allow the availability of hot, prepared meals of more traditional foods when appropriate for the tactical situation. Not only will the rations be more similar to traditional foods, but the eating environment will often be more conducive to greater food intake. Current food technology, packaging, and distribution technology, coupled with efficiently engineered preparation and distribution, should give the combat soldier more acceptable rations in most environments.

Moving in the direction of supplying hot meals whenever possible, including in the field, is an important strategy for overcoming underconsumption and improving morale. However, the MRE may still be used in initial combat operations for varying periods of time to a maximum of 21 days (U.S. Department of the Army, 1995), and data of the type suggested above would be valuable during that initial period. In addition, there are likely to be situations where operational and logistical constraints may require extended use of MREs or related systems. Therefore it seems useful to evaluate those factors that may optimize the MRE system to better meet the nutritional needs of the soldier under these potentially adverse conditions.

RECOMMENDATIONS

The goal of field feeding is to provide sufficient water, food energy, and nutrients to maintain the soldier's hydration status, body weight, and lean body mass. A *field feeding doctrine* should be crafted that incorporates the types and amounts of food offered, issues related to environmental extremes, and actions to be taken with excessive weight loss in the field. From a policy standpoint, the risks that energy deficits will be compounded by uncontrollable events in combat are considerable, and thus any consumption deficits are undesirable. The

TABLE 2-1 Likely Causes of Weight Loss and Potential Impact on Performance[*]

Average Body Weight Loss	Time Period	Likely Cause	Potential Performance Impact
< 3%	24 hours	Inadequate fluid intake	Unlikely
	24 hours–4 days	Energy deficit	Unlikely
> 3% < 10%	Less than 48 hours	Principally inadequate fluid intake	Highly likely, particularly cognitive deficits
	3 days–4 weeks	Energy deficit	Unlikely
> 10%	Less than 48 hours	Inadequate fluid intake	Serious deficits
	3 days–12 weeks	Severe energy deficit	Very likely
	12 weeks or more	Energy deficit	Unlikely

[*] The performance deficits shown in this table will be influenced by (a) the initial body composition of the individual; (b) the speed of weight loss; (c) the composition of the loss (i.e., water and electrolytes, lean body mass, and fat); (d) the presence of trauma, infection, or illness; and (e) the tests being used to measure performance decrements.

guiding principle of this *field feeding doctrine* is that the energy intakes of military personnel during training and combat operations should be adequate to meet their energy expenditures. The level of individual body weight loss should determine the actions to be taken. Suggested criteria for assessing whether energy consumption is adequate to meet energy expenditures for individual soldiers are provided in Table 2-1. Moreover, as suggested by Schnakenberg (IOM, 1995) the appropriate criterion to evaluate whether troops are eating enough of their ration to meet their energy demands should be that the average body weight loss of the test unit does not exceed 3 percent of initial body weight over a period of several weeks.

While underconsumption of operational rations in the training environment is not likely to result in significant reduction in physical or cognitive performance, it may be indicative of a more severe problem when soldiers are under the extreme stresses of impending or actual combat. Therefore steps to minimize underconsumption in training environments may be important when the stress of actual combat operations are imposed.

Since there is evidence that the provision of A or B type rations in training environments does more nearly match energy intake with energy expenditure, it seems important to evaluate the new Army Field Feeding System under operational training environment as early as possible. If this system succeeds in minimizing underconsumption during these training exercises, the focus of research on MREs, T Rations, and other operational rations could be related to evaluating factors that in the short term (3–21 days) may enhance ration consumption or enhance performance in stressful environments.

The Committee on Military Nutrition Research also recommends:

• Even short term deprivation of food intake can lead to performance deficits due to the unpredictable stress of field training, combat situation, hypohydration, and environmental extremes. Every effort should be made to keep soldiers well hydrated to avoid hypohydration-induced anorexia. The goal should be to have individual energy intakes match energy expenditures and thereby provide sufficient food in a manner that encourages soldiers to meet their needs.

• A field feeding doctrine analogous to the highly successful water doctrine, which highlights that food is the fuel of the soldier, should be considered. Such a doctrine will provide guidance to military commanders. In the doctrine an outline of factors that will tend to reduce ration consumption and possible steps to correct these conditions can be useful in helping to ensure that top-notch performance is maintained.

• Because the MRE will continue to be the ration used initially in most military operations, continuing effort should be made to enhance its consumption. Recommended changes include improved individual items including the addition of carry-away snack items, greater variety and enhancements to reduce monotony, improved packaging, better labeling, and creative marketing/training in the importance of the ration and its use.

• Unit commanders should be informed of the potential consequences of weight loss due to dehydration as indicated by a rapid weight loss (2–5 percent in 24–48 hours) or the longer-term effects of underconsumption of rations and should monitor their units to ensure this underconsumption does not adversely affect performance especially during combat. Whenever possible, monitoring should include periodic body weight measurements and other simple anthropometric measures feasible in the field. As a minimum, body weight measures should be done routinely as part of deployment and return activities. Weight losses in the range of 10 percent in operations extending over 4 weeks raise the concern of reduced physical and cognitive performance and have possible health consequences in some of the individuals in the unit.

Since data indicate that the addition of fruit-flavored drinks and flavored shakes with caloric sweeteners to more recent versions of the MRE has led to increases in total energy intake, the CMNR recommends that these items continue to be included in the overall menu program. Further, substitution of existing beverages with artificially-sweetened products may prove counterproductive.

• Unit commanders should be provided guidance as to ways of minimizing the adverse effects of the field environment (e.g., inclement weather, unappetizing local conditions, and lack of congregate meal times) on consumption where possible. This training would improve ration consumption and thus help to minimize performance decrements. The impact of inadequate fluid and food on physiologic function and performance should be emphasized to commanders in light of their importance as role models for increasing soldier food intake.

• Foods provided as snacks can be an important source of energy and other nutrients. Such foods could be provided as part of the MRE or as additional food items.

• A guide should be prepared for commanders in which the impact of various factors involved in food consumption and performance is summarized, based on currently available data. Unit commanders can use such a guide to assist them in making informed decisions concerning the need to improve feeding scenarios during military operations. Such a guide could indicate when changes were needed to avoid possible decrements in unit performance.

• Continued efforts in the development of promotional materials to improve the image of military operational rations, such as the films shown at the workshop, are encouraged. Tied to this effort should be a careful research plan that measures the impact of these materials on soldiers' attitudes.

AREAS FOR FUTURE RESEARCH

The information in this report is primarily derived from data collected during field training exercises. While these observations are important, the impact of the actual exposure to the stresses of combat or impending hostile action is certainly likely to be much greater. Carefully evaluated feedback from soldiers who were deployed in operations such as Vietnam, Desert Storm, and possibly Somalia and Panama could add further insight and realism to the possible extent of underconsumption and influencing factors (e.g., the degree of anxiety, fear, and climatic condition) that would go beyond the information obtained in training exercises. Information on the coping mechanism used by soldiers under these conditions may be useful in considering how to overcome these problems and suggest important areas for research.

The Committee on Military Nutrition Research recognizes the concern that the loss of weight by personnel during training and operations poses to the military. The scientists at the U.S. Army Research Institute of Environmental Medicine (USARIEM) and U.S. Army Natick Research, Development and Engineering Center (NRDEC) have conscientiously followed this issue and conducted carefully planned research programs that have evaluated the impact of food-intake patterns on performance and the factors influencing food intake. The following are suggested by the CMNR as future areas for study that would build on this excellent research base:

• Follow-up interviews with soldiers who participated in Operation Desert Storm that include direct questions about weight loss, food intake, and appetite as well as questions about food items and situational factors would be an important step in interpretation of experimental data. For example, did you lose weight? How much weight? Were you overweight at the start? Why do you think you lost weight? How did you feel about the weight loss? Did you want to lose weight?

• More data on food acceptability under actual rather than simulated field conditions should be collected. This data collection should include both rating scales as well as actual consumption data.

• Focus group research should be carried out with current troops, including women, and with combat veterans with questions directed toward feeding systems in the field including the questions related to MRE packaging, menu items, criticisms, and suggestions for improvement.

• Practical measures should be created to develop, test, and refine a "field feeding doctrine" as described earlier in this report. The food doctrine would be analogous to the successful water doctrine currently in use.

• A simple system should be developed and field tested to monitor body weight and body composition of troops before and after deployment. This system could be used in all field conditions including combat operational training.

• Additional field studies should be conducted that monitor energy intake and energy expenditure using doubly labeled water measurement techniques in temperate and hot environments for comparison with the six existing studies conducted in cold and high-altitude environments. Body composition measures would also be desirable if simple methods were used.

• The relationship between hydration and food intake in military field settings bears additional, carefully designed research.

• The committee believes the existing research on food intake, performance, food item preference, and eating situational factors would first of all benefit from a thorough, careful cross-study integration and interpretation. A multifactorial computerized research model that incorporates the most pertinent findings should then be compiled. This model can be used to assist with the generation of specific hypotheses for future studies, and may be used for selected meta analysis where appropriate.

• Identification of critical and appropriate physical and cognitive tasks, and careful measurement of performance during field operations or recruit training when weight loss is anticipated, would assist in further quantifying the relationship between underconsumption and performance.

• Future field studies should address the question of MRE food item wastage as it relates to specific nutrient intake in relation to energy intake and expenditure.

• The influence of menu variety on intake needs to be tested over a period of time. Carefully designed menu rotation studies that incorporate current understanding of the impact of variety, sensory specific satiety, temporal habituation patterns, energy density, the fat and fiber content of foods, and palatability on intake and body weight could provide directly relevant information.

• A brief study that systematically administered ibuprofen to troops in field exercises could provide information on a potential generalized stress/cytokine/food intake mechanism.

• All future research studies and focus groups should include women and combat veterans where feasible.

The committee commends the development of Kitchen Company Level Field Feeding-Enhanced (KCLFF-E) equipment and the concept of having cooks forward with combat units. After implementation, this system requires follow-up evaluation as to its effectiveness and ways it can be improved.

The CMNR believes that the military services, through their pool of volunteer personnel, offer an excellent and often unique opportunity to generate research data and statistics on the nutrition, health, and stress reduction in service personnel. These findings can be directly applied to improving both the health and the performance of military personnel and those of the general U.S. population.

The Committee on Military Nutrition Research is pleased to participate with the Division of Nutrition, U.S. Army Research Institute of Environmental Medicine, U.S. Army Medical Research and Development Command, in programs related to the nutrition and health of U.S. military personnel. The CMNR hopes that this information will be useful to the U.S. Department of Defense in developing programs that continue to improve the lifetime health and well-being of service personnel.

REFERENCES

Rose, M.S., and D.E. Carlson. 1986. Effects of A Ration meals on body weight during sustained field operations. Technical Report 2-87. Natick, Mass.: U.S. Army Research Institute of Environmental Medicine.

U.S. Department of the Army. 1995. "Revised policy on sole source consumption of Meal, Ready-to-Eat (MRE)." June 21. Washington, D.C.

Vanderveen, J.E., T.H. Allen, G.F. Gee, and R.E. Chapin. 1977. Importance of body fat burden on composition of loss in body mass of men [abstract]. Second International Congress on Obesity, October 23–26, Washington, D.C.

Appendix D

Letter Report: Review of the Revision of the Medical Services Nutrition Allowances, Standards, and Education (AR 40-25, 1985)

Submitted October 1995

INSTITUTE OF MEDICINE
NATIONAL ACADEMY OF SCIENCES
2101 CONSTITUTION AVENUE WASHINGTON, D.C. 20418

FOOD AND NUTRITION BOARD
COMMITTEE ON MILITARY NUTRITION RESEARCH

(202) 334-1737
FAX (202) 334-2316

October 26, 1995

Brig. General R. Zajtchuk
Commanding General
U.S. Army Medical Research and Materiel
   Command (SGRD-ZA)
Fort Detrick
Frederick, MD 21702-5012

Dear General Zajtchuk:

At the specific request of the COL Eldon W. Askew, Ph.D., (former) Chief, Military Nutrition Division, U.S. Army Research Institute of Environmental Medicine (USARIEM) and Grant Officer Representative of the U.S. Army Medical Research and Materiel Command (USAMRMC, the Command) for Grant No. DAMD17-92-J-2003 to the National Academy of Sciences for support of the Food and Nutrition Board's (FNB) Committee on Military Nutrition Research (CMNR), members of the CMNR met in Washington, D.C. on February 1, 1994. A partial purpose of this meeting was to provide additional scientific guidance to the staff of the Office of the Surgeon General, Department of the Army (OTSG, DA) in reviewing their latest revision of the Medical Services Nutrition Allowances, Standards, and Education (AR 40-25, 1985). This document is a Joint Army, Navy and Air Force Regulation for which the OTSG, DA is identified as the DoD Executive Agent for Nutrition and has responsibility for drafting revisions and coordinating changes with the responsible offices in the other Services. The CMNR was requested to perform this review as part of its task to provide scientific support to USARIEM, which has the mission to perform military nutrition and related research.

Prior to the meeting, the CMNR reviewed (1) Army Regulation 40-25/Naval Command Medical Instruction 10110.1/Air Force Regulation 160-95, "Nutrition Allowances, Standards, and Education," (AR 40-25, 1985); and (2) the proposed revision submitted by COL Karen Fridlund (see Attachment

97

II–henceforth called AR 40-25REV), (former) Chief Dietitian, Office of the Surgeon General, Department of the Army.

The Committee on Military Nutrition Research's role at the meeting was to evaluate, comment upon, and make specific recommendations for changes in the entire revised document with special attention to Chapter 2, "Nutritional Allowances and Standards," that includes the Military Recommended Dietary Allowances (MRDAs), Estimated Safe and Adequate Daily Dietary Intakes, and Nutrient Standards for Operational and Restricted Rations as they reflect changes in the latest version of the *Recommended Dietary Allowances* (RDAs), published by the Food and Nutrition Board (NRC, 1989b) and other relevant national policy statements on nutrition and health such as the *Surgeon General's Report on Nutrition and Health* (DHHS, 1988) and the *Diet and Health* report (NRC, 1989a). This task was not in the original plan of work for the committee as part of Grant DAMD17-92-J-2003 from the U.S. Army, which ended on May 31, 1994. The CMNR has made completion of this report its highest priority under its new grant DAMD17-94-J-4046 which was initiated on November 1, 1994. A list of committee members present at the initial meeting and the current committee membership roster are included as Attachment A.

This report of the CMNR has been reviewed in accordance with National Research Council (NRC) guidelines by a separate anonymous scientific review panel. This report is thus based on executive session discussions by the committee and is a thoughtfully developed presentation incorporating the scientific opinion of the CMNR and comments of the anonymous peer review panel of the NRC.

This letter contains a summary of the Committee on Military Nutrition Research's evaluation of AR 40-25REV and the Committee recommendations. There are three attachments with this letter: Attachment I lists the members of the Committee on Military Nutrition Research (CMNR) who participated in this review; Attachment II is AR 40-25REV as presented to the Committee for review; and Attachment III contains an elaboration of the recommendations and comments in this letter.

Attachment III is organized into four sections. First, there are more detailed explanations of the recommendations and comments that pertain to the MRDAs in general that are included here. Second, there is a listing of general comments regarding the text of AR 40-25REV that was reviewed by the CMNR. Third, there are specific comments directed to questions or concerns that the CMNR believe need to be addressed before publication of the revision. To assist with clear interpretation of the specific comments, a reference version of AR 40-25REV has been included in Attachment III (henceforth called AR 40-25REF). The line numbers cited in the specific comments below refer to AR 40-25REF. Fourth, the CMNR and the anonymous reviewers of this report have suggested wording changes for the text of AR 40-25REV. These have been made directly in the text of AR 40-25REF. The suggested wording for removal has been indicated by ~~cross-out~~ and the recommended new wording indicated by highlighting; these suggested changes are not discussed in any detail in the text of the report.

RECOMMENDATIONS AND COMMENTS REGARDING
AR 40-25REV

On the basis of past reviews of AR 40-25, recent reviews of military rations and ration developments, recent workshops on nutrient requirements for military personnel in environmental extremes, and committee deliberations regarding the present version of AR 40-25REV, the CMNR presents the following recommendations to the U.S. Army Medical Research and Materiel Command (USAMRMC) regarding AR 40-25REV. The CMNR believes that the comments and recommendations in this report are also of significance to those responsible for establishing nutritional policy for the DoD in the Office of The Surgeon General, Department of the Army, as well as those responsible for the planning and procurement of military rations. The Committee particularly wants to call the attention of those individuals to Sections B and C in Attachment III.

• The staffs of OTSG, DA and USAMRMC are urged to review whether there continues to be a need to maintain separate MRDAs (specifically sections 2.1, 2.2, 2.4, and 2.5, which are derived from the RDAs), in light of existing information that has been developed by the IOM, DHHS, and other organizations for the general population.

• The CMNR recommends that Table 2-3 on nutritional standards for operational and restricted rations be retained and that the narrative accompanying the table values (section 2.3) explain clearly how the reference values were derived.

• If it is determined by the OTSG, DA that the military version of the RDAs (sections 2.1, 2.2, 2.4, and 2.5) is to be maintained, the CMNR recommends that serious consideration be given to the future mechanism for development of these sections as well as the nutrient standards for operational or restricted rations (section 2.3). The CMNR cannot identify a group within the existing DoD structure with a sufficient depth and breadth of expertise to develop these recommendations. There is a critical need for a group of individuals who are familiar with the development of RDAs to assist in the derivation of the MRDAs as well as the nutritional standards.

• The CMNR further recommends that, if it continues to be the view of the OTSG, DA that the MRDAS and nutritional standards for operational and restricted rations are needed, then:

• the scientific expertise at USARIEM should be involved in the future in the development of such standards to assure consideration of the findings of research conducted by the Military Nutrition Division at USARIEM;

• a joint review by nutritionists/dietitians from each of the Services is desirable to assure consideration of issues of special concern to each of the branches of the military, in the development of these MRDAs and standards since they are applicable to the Army, Air Force, and Navy; and

• timely consideration by the military of dietary recommendations developed by the Food and Nutrition Board should occur as new versions are released.

CONCLUSIONS

It is the view of the CMNR that there does not appear to be a scientific basis to have distinct military recommended dietary allowances for individuals performing duties in normal peacetime military operations and non-field conditions. However, since the MRDAs have an extensive history of use by the military in areas such as menu planning and procurement of military rations, the Committee recognizes that they may serve an essential purpose beyond that usually identified with the RDAs. In addition, nutritional standards for the development and procurement of operational and restricted rations are necessary to assure that the issued rations meet the needs of service men and women whose entire diet while under simulated or actual combat conditions may consist of the issued rations for extended periods of time, such as experienced during Operation Desert Shield/Storm and during peace-keeping operations in Somalia and Haiti.

The CMNR is pleased to provide this review as part of its continuing response to the U.S. Army Medical Research and Materiel Command. The Committee always welcomes comments and suggestions from you or your staff regarding how these reports can better serve the purpose of the Army.

Sincerely,

Robert O. Nesheim, Ph.D.
Chairman, Committee on Military
Nutrition Research

Enclosures

cc: F. Hagge
     H. Lieberman

K. Shine
K. Hein
A. Yates
B. Marriott

REFERENCES

AR 40-25. 1985. *See* U.S. Departments of the Army, the Navy, and the Air Force.

NRC (National Research Council). 1989a. Diet and Health: Implication for Reducing Chronic Disease Risk. A report of the Committee on Diet and Health, Food and Nutrition Board, Commission on Life Sciences. Washington, D.C.: National Academy Press.

NRC. 1989b. Recommended Dietary Allowances, 10th ed. A report of the Subcommittee on the Tenth Edition of the RDAs, Food and Nutrition Board, Commission on Life Sciences. Washington, D.C.: National Academy Press.

U.S. Departments of the Army, the Navy, and the Air Force. 1985. Army Regulation 40-25/Naval Command Medical Instruction 10110.1/Air Force Regulation 160-95. "Nutrition Allowances, Standards, and Education." May 15. Washington, D.C.

Attachment I

COMMITTEE ON MILITARY NUTRITION RESEARCH ROSTER

Robert O. Nesheim, Ph.D. (Chair)
28009 Mesa de Tierra
Salinas, CA 93908
(408) 484-9296 FAX (408) 484-1903

William R. Beisel, M.D.
Adjunct Professor, Department of
   Immunology and Infectious Diseases
Johns Hopkins School of Hygiene and
   Public Health
Baltimore, MD 21205
Mailing address: 8210 Ridgelea
Frederick, MD 21702
(301) 662-2745

Gail E. Butterfield, Ph.D.
Director, Nutrition Studies
Palo Alto Veterans Affairs Health Care
   System(GRECC/182-B)
Visiting Associate Professor, Program in
   Human Biology, Stanford University
3801 Miranda Avenue
Palo Alto, CA 94304
(415) 493-5000 Ex 64577 or 63289
FAX (415) 855-9437

John D. Fernstrom, Ph.D.
Professor of Psychiatry, Pharmacology
   and Neuroscience
University of Pittsburgh School of
   Medicine
Western Psychiatric Institute and Clinic
3811 O'Hara Street, Room 1620
Pittsburgh, PA 15213
(412) 624-2032 FAX (412) 624-3696
FERNSTRO+@PITT.EDU

G. Richard Jansen, Ph.D.
Professor Emeritus, Department of Food
   Science and Human Nutrition
Colorado State University
Gifford Bldg., Room 205
Fort Collins, CO 80523
(970) 484-3212 FAX (970) 491-7252

Robin B. Kanarek, Ph.D.
Professor of Psychology
Department of Psychology
Tufts University
490 Boston Avenue
Medford, MA 02155
(617) 628-5000 Ext. 5902
FAX (617) 627-3178
RKANAREK@PEARL.TUFTS.EDU

Orville A. Levander, Ph.D.
Research Leader
Nutrient Requirements and Functions
   Laboratory
U.S. Department of Agriculture
ARS, BHNRC, Building 307, Room 117
Beltsville, MD 20705
(301) 504-8351 FAX (301) 504-9062

Gilbert A. Leveille, Ph.D.
Vice President
Research and Technical Services
Nabisco Foods Group
200 DeForest Avenue, P.O. Box 1944
East Hanover, NJ 07936-1944
(201) 503-4770 FAX (201) 515-9229

John E. Vanderveen, Ph.D.
Director, Office of Plant and Dairy Foods
   and Beverages
Food and Drug Administration
200 C Street, SW
Washington, DC 20204
(202) 205-4064 FAX (202) 205-4422

Douglas W. Wilmore, M.D.
Frank Sawyer Professor
Department of Surgery
Brigham and Women's Hospital
Boston, MA 02115
(617) 732-5280 FAX (617) 732-5506

Food and Nutrition Board Liaison to Committee:

Johanna T. Dwyer, D.Sc., R.D.
Director, Frances Stern Nutrition Center
Professor, Department of Medicine
Tufts Medical School and New England
    Medical Center
750 Washington Street, Box #783
Boston, MA 02111
(617) 636-5273 FAX (617) 636-8325

**U.S. Army Grant Officer
Representative:**

Harris R. Lieberman, Ph.D.
Chief, Military Nutrition Division
Occupational Heath and Performance
    Directorate
USARIEM
ATTN: MCMR-UE-OPN
Natick, MA 01760-5007
(508) 233-4856 FAX (508) 651-4195
(508) 233-4859 (Secretary)

NRC Staff:

Bernadette M. Marriott, Ph.D.
Study Director

Sydne J. Carlson, Ph.D.
Program Officer

Susan M. Knasiak
Research Assistant

Donna F. Allen
Project Assistant
(202) 334-1737 FAX (202) 334-2316

COMMITTEE ON MILITARY NUTRITION RESEARCH ROSTER
(former committee, January 1994)

Robert O. Nesheim, Ph.D. (Chair)
28009 Mesa de Tierra
Salinas, CA 93908
(408) 484-9296 FAX (408) 484-1903

Richard L. Atkinson, M.D.
Professor of Medicine and Nutritional
  Sciences
University of Wisconsin-Madison
1415 Linden Drive, Nutritional Sciences
  Bldg.
Madison, WI 53706
(608) 262-2727 FAX (608) 262-5860

William R. Beisel, M.D.
Adjunct Professor, Department of
  Immunology and Infectious Diseases
Johns Hopkins School of Hygiene and
  Public Health
Baltimore, MD 21205
Mailing address: 8210 Ridgelea
Frederick, MD 21702
(301) 662-2745

Gail E. Butterfield, Ph.D.
Stanford University School of Medicine
Division of Endocrinology, Gerontology,
  and Metabolism
Geriatric Research, Education, and
  Clinical Center
VA Medical Center (GRECC/182-B)
3801 Miranda Avenue
Palo Alto, CA 94304
(415) 493-5000 FAX (415) 855-9437

John D. Fernstrom, Ph.D.
Professor of Psychiatry, Pharmacology
  and Neuroscience
University of Pittsburgh School of
  Medicine
Western Psychiatric Institute and Clinic
3811 O'Hara Street, Room 1620
Pittsburgh, PA 15213
(412) 624-2032 FAX (412) 624-3696

Joël A. Grinker, Ph.D.
Professor, Pediatrics and Communicable
  Diseases
Program in Human Nutrition
School of Public Health
University of Michigan
1420 Washington Heights - M5170
Ann Arbor, MI 48109
(313) 764-5270 FAX (313) 763-5455

G. Richard Jansen, Ph.D.
Professor Emeritus, Department of Food
  Science and Human Nutrition
Colorado State University
Gifford Bldg., Room 205
Fort Collins, CO 80523
(303) 484-3212 FAX (303) 491-7252

Orville A. Levander, Ph.D.
Vitamin and Mineral Nutrition
  Laboratory
USDA, ARS, BHNRC
Building 307, Room 117
Beltsville, MD 20705
(301) 504-8351 FAX (301) 504-9062

Gilbert A. Leveille, Ph.D.
Vice President
Research and Technical Services
Nabisco Foods Group
200 DeForest Avenue
P.O. Box 1944
East Hanover, NJ 07936-1944
(201) 503-4770 FAX (201) 515-9229

John E. Vanderveen, Ph.D.
Director, Office of Plant and Dairy Foods
  and Beverages
Food and Drug Administration
200 C Street, SW
Washington, DC 20204
(202) 205-4064 FAX (202) 205-4594

Food and Nutrition Board Liaison to Committee:

Johanna T. Dwyer, D.Sc., R.D.
Professor, Department of Medicine,
    Tufts Medical School and New
    England Medical Center
Director, Frances Stern Nutrition Center
750 Washington Street, Box #783
Boston, MA 02111
(617) 956-5273 FAX (617) 524-1252

U.S. Army Grant Officer Representative:

Dr. James A. Vogel
Director, Occupational Health and
    Performance Directorate
USARIEM
ATTN: SGRD-UE-OPN
Natick, MA 01760-5007
(508) 651-4800 FAX (508) 651-5833
FAX AV 256-5298

NRC Staff:

Bernadette M. Marriott, Ph.D.
Program Director

Donna F. Allen
Project Assistant

(202) 334-1737 FAX (202) 334-2316

Attachment III

CMNR ELABORATION OF RECOMMENDATIONS AND COMMENTS REGARDING AR40-25 REV

A. CMNR RECOMMENDATIONS AND COMMENTS REGARDING THE MRDAS: FURTHER EXPLANATION

The major recommendations as presented in the letter are underlined and followed by additional explanation.

• The staffs of OTSG, DA and USAMRMC are urged to review whether there continues to be a need to maintain separate MRDAs (specifically sections 2.1, 2.2, 2.4, and 2.5, which are derived from the RDAs), in light of existing information that has been developed by the IOM, DHHS, and other organizations for the general population. This information is primarily found in two reports from the Food and Nutrition Board, the *Recommended Dietary Allowances* (RDAs), Tenth Edition (NRC, 1989b) and the *Diet and Health* report (NRC, 1989a), in the U.S. Department of Health and Human Services (DHHS) report, the *Surgeon General's Report on Nutrition and Health* (1988), in the U.S. Department of Agriculture (USDA) and DHHS report, *Dietary Guidelines for Americans* (USDA and DHHS, 1990), and in the recent USDA *Report of the Dietary Guidelines Advisory Committee on the Dietary Guidelines for Americans, 1995* (USDA, 1995). The MRDAs provide reference values for the development of the Master Menu, military rations, and for procurement of food for healthy active military personnel. They are adaptations of the RDAs and are defined as the "...daily essential nutrient intake levels presently considered to meet the known nutritional needs of practically all 17- to 50-year old, moderately active military personnel" (AR 40-25, 1985). The MRDAs have been based on the RDAs but modified to reflect the assumptions of additional energy requirements of active military personnel, differing nutrient requirements for work in environmental extremes, and amounts to achieve a palatable diet. It was assumed, in addition, that military personnel differed significantly from the general American population in terms of age, fitness, body composition, as well as activity. The CMNR questions whether the military population in the 1990s varies significantly from the American population in ways that would not be addressed within the framework of the previously mentioned nutritional and dietary guidelines. Therefore, the CMNR suggests that the Army consider adopting the RDAs and *Dietary Guidelines for Americans*, and modifying the RDAs only for nutrients where sufficient scientific evidence exists to justify a change due to energy expenditure or environmental demands typical for moderately active personnel.

• The CMNR recommends that Table 2-3 on nutritional standards for operational and restricted rations be retained and that the narrative accompanying the table values (section 2.3) explain clearly how the reference values were derived. Operational and restricted rations are designed to provide the total nutrition for soldiers in combat, in highly specific settings, and usually for a specified time period. As such the expected energy expenditure and nutritional needs of military personnel under these conditions can be expected to vary significantly from the normal requirements of moderately active individuals. These standards are also used by ration planners in the development and procurement of operational rations where it is necessary to provide the entire diet for the active duty soldier over sustained operations.

• <u>If it is determined by the OTSG, DA that the military version of the RDAs (sections 2.1, 2.2, 2.4, and 2.5) is to be maintained, the CMNR recommends that serious consideration be given to the future mechanism for development of these sections as well as the nutrient standards for operational or restricted rations (section 2.3). The CMNR cannot identify a group within the existing DoD structure with a sufficient depth and breadth of expertise to develop these recommendations. There is a critical need for a group of individuals who are familiar with the development of RDAs to assist in the derivation of the MRDAs as well as the nutritional standards.</u> The RDAs are developed on a periodic basis by a panel of scientific experts, convened by the Food and Nutrition Board, who carefully review the existing scientific information, consult extensively with scientific colleagues, and prepare a document that then is reviewed both by the Food and Nutrition Board members and anonymous peers. The CMNR believes that the military dietary recommendations, as the basis for nutritional information for the United States Armed Forces, similarly require the careful development by scientific experts. The CMNR can serve as a peer review panel for the MRDAs but since it is constituted to deal with a wide variety of issues in nutrition, health, and performance, it may not have the scientific depth in each nutrient to develop specific military recommendations where needed. Therefore, the CMNR recommends that, when the MRDAs are to be revised (usually as a result of a revision of the RDAs or specific consideration of operational ration requirements), the Army consider supporting the review through the CMNR. In this manner the necessary scientific expertise can be assembled to address the areas needing in-depth evaluation—much as is currently done through the CMNR when it is asked to review such questions as nutrition in hot environments and the effects of cold and altitude on nutritional needs. In this task the group may require full access to a liaison panel of tri-service nutritionists/dietitians as well as military nutrition researchers from USARIEM who can provide the necessary and relevant military information.

B. GENERAL COMMENTS ON AR 40-25REV

In addition to the recommendations presented above, the CMNR presents eleven general comments about AR 40-25REV for the consideration of the Army.

• It is expected that the RDAs will begin to undergo revision in 1995. It is anticipated that there will be significant changes in the conceptual basis and format of the new recommendations (see How Should the Recommended Dietary Allowances Be Revised? IOM, 1994b). It would be highly desirable to harmonize AR 40-25 with the anticipated changes in the RDAs. Due to these anticipated changes in the RDAs, AR 40-25 needs to include a clear, concise rationale on a nutrient-by-nutrient basis for derivation of the values. This could be accomplished by a clearly footnoted table or with more detailed information in the text for each nutrient. At present, as noted in the specific comments below, there are inconsistencies between the RDAs and AR 40-25REV that are not clearly explained in the text or tables.

• A section needs to be added discussing the rationale behind and the derivation of the values for the Operational and Restricted Rations.

• Although the CMNR recognizes that 99.6 percent of the military population is between the ages of 17 and 50 years, the CMNR believes the regulation would be enhanced for the user by additional text that comments on energy and energy-based nutrient values that change with age.

• The CMNR strongly recommends that allowances for pregnancy and lactation be indicated in AR 40-25REV tables and clearly explained in the text. The CMNR recognizes that at this time women comprise only 12 percent of military personnel. The last version of AR 40-25 will have been in effect without revision for 10 years before the new revision is published. On this basis, within the next time cycle of regulation revision, the CMNR envisions the potential for a significant increase in the number of women in military service.

• There are numerous inconsistencies in the recommended fluid intake and electrolyte values and accompanying text. The CMNR also recommends a careful and thorough evaluation of this section of AR 40-25 in relation to recommendations in the RDAs (NRC, 1989b), the Surgeon General's Report on Nutrition and Health (DHHS, 1988), and the Diet and Health report (NRC, 1989a). The CMNR has reviewed different aspects of this issue for the DoD in several recent reports (see for example: Military Nutrition Initiatives, IOM,

1991a; Fluid Replacement and Heat Stress, IOM [3 printings] 1991b, 1992b, 1994a; Nutritional Needs in Hot Environments, IOM, 1993).

• The word requirement is used incorrectly in several places in the text; the word allowance should be substituted. The definition of a requirement for an adult is

"...with an amount (of a nutrient [Ed.])that will maintain body weight and prevent depletion of the nutrient from the body, as judged by balance studies and maintenance of acceptable blood and tissue concentrations. For certain nutrients, the requirement may be the amount that will prevent failure of a specific function or the development of specific deficiency signs–an amount that may differ greatly from that required to maintain body stores" (NRC, 1989b, p. 11).

These specific instances are marked in AR 40-25REF. To clarify this point for users of the AR 40-25REV, the CMNR further suggests that the terms *requirement, recommendations*, and *allowances* be added to the glossary of AR 40-25REV.

• There are many numerical inconsistencies throughout AR 40-25REV that appear to result from no standard way of numerical "rounding" after calculations are performed. An approach to numerical rounding is stated in the initial chapters of most statistical textbooks and should be applied to these calculations.

• There is no information regarding the derivation of the value for Phosphorus levels in Tables 2-1 or 2-3. The information included in the 1985 document included discussion of the Ca:P ratio. This was not included here. Consideration also should be given to adding guidance in Chapter 3 regarding life-long high intakes of high phosphorus-containing soft drinks.

• All of the nutrients that are included in Table 2-1 are not discussed in the text. To make the discussion complete, all nutrients should be included in the discussion in section 2-5.

• Throughout the document there is a recurring problem of putting two thoughts together; even though they are related, the way they are presented causes confusion. To mention but a few examples, page 47 lines 633-634, "Most health professionals recommend a diet containing less total fat, saturated fat and cholesterol". It appears that the point trying to be made is that many health professionals suggest that a diet low in fat, saturated fat and cholesterol is healthy. Another example occurs on page 49 lines 661-663, "Complex carbohydrates are more nutrient dense and contain greater amounts of dietary fiber than foods high in simple carbohydrates such as sweets, cakes, candy, sugar-sweetened beverages, etc." It appears that the point trying to be communicated is that foods containing complex carbohydrates are typically more nutrient dense than those containing simple carbohydrates. Complex carbohydrates may also be a source of dietary fiber. Special attention needs to be placed on reviewing the document for this problem.

• The reference format is inconsistent throughout the document. Text references should either include authors and year or title, author, and year, or be cited numerically. All references should be as complete as possible. All references cited in the text must be cross checked and included in the reference list. Many references that are currently in the text are not included in the reference list. The entire draft regulation requires thorough proofreading and the use of a professional copy editor to address general editing problems of this nature as well as the use of correct English, spelling (dietitian should replace dietician) and scientific abbreviations; for example "calorie" should be replaced with kcal as a measurement of energy throughout the text.

C. SPECIFIC COMMENTS REGARDING AR 40-25REV

The comments below are indicated by Section, and where appropriate, by line number in AR 40-25REF that follows.

Chapter 1

1-1. No comments.

1-2. References. The CMNR recommends that the following references be added as related references: Nutrition During Pregnancy (IOM, 1990); Nutrition During Lactation (IOM, 1991c); Nutrition During Pregnancy and Lactation: An Implementation Guide ((IOM, 1992c); Body Composition and Physical Performance (IOM, 1992a); Military Nutrition Initiatives (IOM, 1991a); and Nutritional Needs in Hot Environments (IOM, 1993). In addition it is not clear what is meant by "required publications". Rationale should be provided to indicate by whom and for what these references are required.

1-3. See suggested changes in glossary of AR 40-25REF.

1-4a. The CMNR concurs with the inclusion of simulated combat conditions as a situation under which MRDAs must be met.
1-4a. The CMNR strongly supports the maintenance of military nutrition research capability through the U.S. Army Medical Research and Materiel

Command, particularly through utilizing the combined support available at the U.S. Army Research Institute of Environmental Medicine (USARIEM) facilities located in Natick, Massachusetts.

1.4a. See suggested wording changes in AR 40-25REF.

1-4b. No comments.

Chapter 2

2-1a. The wording throughout this section was not clear. See suggested changes in AR 40-25REF.

   Line 111. After stating that the MRDAs are listed in Table 2-1, it would be helpful to add that the values are expressed in terms of "reference individuals" for each gender. See the text pertaining to reference individuals in the National Research Council's Recommended Dietary Allowances, 10th Edition (pp. 14-15). The RDA values are the actual medians of height and weight for the U.S. population of the designated age and gender, as reported in the second National Health and Nutrition Examination Survey (NHANES II).

2-1b. No comments.

2-1c. Lines 121-126. This statement does not match the calculated values in Table 2-1 because the energy values in the table assume moderate to heavy physical activity. Please consider revising text or table values for consistency.

2-1d. No comments.

2-2. See suggested wording changes in AR 40-25REF.

2-3a-b. See suggested wording changes in AR 40-25REF.

2-3d. The CMNR is unable to comment on this section since it has not reviewed the Food Packet, Survival, Abandon Ship Survival Ration, or the Aircraft/Life Raft Ration.

2-3d. See suggested wording changes in AR 40-25REF.

2-4. It is suggested that the current section 2-4c. Physical Activity would be more appropriately placed as section 2-4b; with the present section 2-4b. Body Size moved to become section 2-4c.

2-4a. See suggested wording changes in AR 40-25REF.

2-4b. See suggested wording changes in AR 40-25REF.

   Lines 193-196. These last sentences need to be changed as shown in the text or a longer rationale needs to be provided.

2-4c. See suggested wording changes in AR 40-25REF. The values here contradict those described in Section 2-1c. In addition, there appears to be confusion within the table and between the table and text regarding energy recommendations. There is considerable inconsistency. Many of the values in

Table 2-1 were calculated using the *average* MRDA value for energy, which pertains to those who engage, by the table definitions, in *moderate to heavy activity*. All MRDA values need to be recalculated based on consistent energy recommendations. Table 2-1, would be more readily understood if a supporting table was generated that provided a listing of typical military activities and classified them as light, moderate, heavy and very heavy physical activity.

2-4d. See suggested wording changes in AR 40-25REF.

2-4d. (1) See suggested wording changes in AR 40-25REF.

2-4d. (2) See suggested wording changes in AR 40-25REF.

Line 232. The sentence that begins "Beyond 30 degrees..." is very specific. To include this level of specificity in the text requires that a solid scientific reference be cited.

Line 236. It is suggested that the following sentence be added at the end of this paragraph and the implications considered carefully: "This requirement, when computed, results in 4,370 kcal/day for the reference moderately active military man; 3,415 kcal/day for the military woman."

2-4d. (3) The CMNR suggests that this section be *replaced* by the following: "Altitude: Energy requirements for high-altitude operations, greater than 10,000 ft (3,050 m) are increased due to: (1) 15% elevation in basal metabolism, (2) performance of physical activities over rugged terrain, and (3) physiological response to cold. Total energy requirements for individuals performing strenuous work at altitude may reach 6,000 kcal/d. The loss of appetite that occurs at high altitude coupled with this increased need makes obtaining sufficient energy to maintain lean body mass very difficult to attain without conscious effort and may require a disciplined food and water intake program." (Keep last sentence in this section. There is little evidence that chronic altitude exposure increases the requirement for any specific nutrients other than carbohydrate and water.)

2-4d. (4) See suggested wording changes in AR 40-25REF.

2-5a. See suggested wording changes in AR 40-25REF.

2-5b. The CMNR wishes to congratulate the Army on its education programs that were successful in reducing fat intake in garrison from a range of 41.8 to 48.6% to 34.0 to 38.4% (IOM, 1991a, p. 95) and suggests additional studies that would similarly measure the impact of nutrition education initiatives. The statement in AR 40-25REV regarding saturated fats in the diet is modeled after the statement in the 1989 edition of the RDAs, but the CMNR cautions that this approach may warrant consideration in light of recent changes in the *Dietary Guidelines for Americans* and pending changes in the RDAs.

Lines 264-269. Does this refer to shipboard and garrison only? Please clarify.

2-5c. "Complex carbohydrates are more nutrient dense..." with regard to what? relative to vitamins and minerals? This section is not clear. Also see suggested wording changes in AR 40-25REF.

2-5d. See suggested wording changes in AR 40-25REF. Although low fat dairy products are healthier, their calcium content is not dramatically different.

2-5e. Lines 296-299. The CMNR suggests that the last two sentences of section 2-5e be removed because the current RDAs do not indicate a need for supplementation for lower energy intake levels in women.

2-5f. This statement focuses entirely on salt as a source of iodine. Other sources should be mentioned so there will not be contradictions with other sections of AR 40-25REV where a reduction in salt intake is recommended.

2-5g. See suggested wording changes in AR 40-25REF.

2-5h. (1) See suggested wording changes in AR 40-25REF. It is suggested for clarity that the following be added **after line 315**: "The MRDAs for sodium are based on an average level of energy expenditure (3,600 kcal/day for men; 2,500 kcal/day for women). The table values, 5,600 mg/day for men and 3,900 mg/day for women, are the average values that were calculated using the range 1,400-1,700 mg sodium/1,000 kcal (rounded to the nearest 50 mg increment)." The CMNR further notes that there is no scientific reference provided for the basis of the MRDA value for sodium.

2-5h. (2) See suggested wording changes in AR 40-25REF. The CMNR advises that both "discretionary" and "non-discretionary" sodium intake should be defined in the glossary. Also note that the citation of the CMNR Activity Report as a reference is inaccurate. There is no identifiable reference in this report to salt tablets. In addition, the CMNR Activity Reports are summaries of previous reports and the correct citation would be the original report.

2-5i. Water. See suggested wording changes in AR 40-25REF.

Lines 330-333. This statement is referenced erroneously to the CMNR report, *Nutritional Needs in Hot Environments* (IOM, 1993). Perhaps this statement could be supported through a derivation from Carl Gisolfi's chapter in that report, but this does not appear to be the case. For CMNR reports, the authored chapters must be cited by the author's name and year and referenced as a titled chapter in the report. The CMNR report can only be cited as a reference if the material is based on chapters 1 and 2 that were written by the committee. This fact is clearly stated in each CMNR report.

NOTE: There is something wrong with the assumptions with respect to water. See calculations below for what recommendations under "water" appear to suggest.

1. Assume 1 ml water/kcal as a reasonable basis.

2. Assume average energy expenditures as indicated in Table 2-1. Therefore: for men 3.6 L and for women 2.5 L.

3. Assume in hot climates water need increases by 1.5-2 times, then

    5.4-7.2 L for men   3.75-5.0 L for women

4. Assume in addition, if heavy work is done fluid needs increase 3 fold so, 3.6 x 3 = or 2.5 x 3 =

    10.8 L for men   7.5 L for women

5. Assume if all of the above are true, and the soldier arrives at high altitude, that 3-4 liters additional are suggested, plus 200-300 g of carbohydrate

    13.8-17.8 L for men   10.5-11.5 L for women

6. Assume an additional 4 liters over the 3-4 liters additional in step 5. if the individual is in an engine room or MOPP4 garments

    14.8 L for men   11.5 L for women

NOTE: These recommendations result in different levels, e.g., 3.6 L and 2.5 L, for temperate climates than the 6 L suggested at the end of the AR 40-25REV text in section 2-5i.Water; using average energy intakes as stated in the regulation.

Also, the rationale or derivation of values for Arctic climates of 8 L at line 346 is not provided at all and needs to be. Basically, increased fluid intake for active personnel in the cold is dependent on sweating plus excessive respiratory water loss because of the low ambient vapor pressure. The committee has deleted this section in AR 40-25REF since there is no reference cited.

The calculations for water needs for hot environments to arrive at the value of 12 L on line 346 also are not clear. If we took assumption 3 above and added assumption 6, the result would be 9.4-11.2 L for men and 7.75-9.0 L for women, *not* 12 L. Finally, it is not clear to what base figure a 4 L per day increment for working in a hot engine room or MOPP4 suit should be added? Is it 1 ml/kcal plus adjustments for hot climate of 1.5-2 times, or 3 times for hot climate plus work? The MOPP4 garments should be included in this discussion as well as a definition of this term.

Please note again that the method of citing scientific references is inconsistent and scientifically inaccurate. *Nutrition in Exercise and Sport* is an edited volume. Any reference to material from this book needs to be cited by the names of the authors of the chapter in which the material is found and the publication year. The CMNR did not read this book to try to verify this information in **lines 333 to 339** and therefore cannot make any comment on this high altitude recommendation for additional fluid and carbohydrate. Rewording has been suggested for readability.

2-5j. Supplemental beverages. See suggested wording changes in AR 40-25REF.

Lines 362-364. "With normal fluid and food intake, carbohydrate and electrolyte ~~balance~~ losses due to stress may be restored..." This is not clear; restored by what?

Lines 364-366. Inaccurate reference citation to the *CMNR Activity Report, 1986-1992.* This is a summary report of activities. Citations must be attributed to the original report or authored chapters in original reports.

Lines 368-371. This is an inaccurate reference citation to the report, *Nutritional Needs in Hot Environments.* The correct report has been cited in the text.

Lines 373-376. See comment above regarding the use of the title of an edited volume as a reference and revise to provide a specific scientifically accurate reference.

Specific Comments on Table 2-1 See suggested wording changes in AR 40-25REF.

Please state the reference weight standard in the table (e.g., 78 kg, 61 kg).

Energy: Use a standard figure for all calculations. The committee found it confusing to have it stated that moderate activity levels were selected, when, in fact, many of the values in AR 40-25REV were calculated using the higher AVG Energy. Thus, 3,150 and 2,250 are not the base (e.g., moderate activity for men and women). All AR 40-25REV values should be calculated using the same energy needs. Footnotes are needed to explain many values in the table. Below are the calculations attempted by the CMNR to derive the table values. This type of information must be added to the text *and* footnoted in Table 2-1 for clarity.

Protein: The recommended allowance for reference protein is 0.75 g/kg and 0.8 g/kg is the recommended dietary allowance for U.S. Dietary Protein (RDAs, NRC, 1989b). A value that takes into account newer studies suggesting higher values with physical activity is 1.5 g/kg. The mid-point of this range is used to calculate a reference weight for men of 78 kg and reference weight for women of 61 kg.

Thiamin (B^1): This calculation is based on 0.5 mg/1,000 kcal (RDAs, NRC, 1989b) assuming AVG Energy values, therefore 1.8 mg (men), and 1.25 mg or 1.3 mg, (women).

Riboflavin: The MRDA value is based on 0.6 mg per 1,000 kcal (RDAs, NRC, 1989a) using AVG Energy values, therefore 2.16 or 2.2 mg (men) and 1.3 mg (women).

Niacin: The RDA appears to be different from the value in AR 40-25REV. Why? Possible calculation is 6.6 NE/1,000 kcal; therefore 16.5 or 17 mg.

Vitamin B⁶: Typographical error—It should read B_6^9 not B-9. In footnote #9, explicitly state the equation from the 1989 RDA to show how the AR 40-25REV value is calculated.

Folic Acid: The folic acid value was calculated using 78 kg reference weight for men and 3 µg/kg body weight (RDAs, NRC, 1989b). The value for women correctly differs from the RDA because of a more recent directive from the U.S. Public Health Service; this directive should be cited.

Sodium: See previous comments. It is unclear how the values 5,600 and 3,900 mg were derived if the value of 1.0 mg/kcal was used as the basis for the calculation. Please recalculate these values and present clear rationales for their calculation. Clearly the footnote is incorrect. In addition, these are not sodium requirements but rather recommendations.

NOTE: It is not clear how the sodium recommendation was derived. The 1989 RDAs only provide a *minimum* recommendation.

- On the basis of AVG Energy, sodium recommendation would be:
  Men   3,600 mg
  Women   2,500 mg

- If 1,400-1,700 mg Na/1,000 kcal, then
  Men = 5,040-6,120 mg for 3,600 kcal AVG Energy
  Women = 3,500-4,250 mg for 2,500 kcal AVG Energy
  or a midpoint of 3,875. These do not agree with the RDAs.

Line 436. The reference is cited incorrectly. The author and year of publication should be cited in the text. Then the full citation should be included in the reference list. This reference citation cannot be understood as it presently is written.

Line 443. This reference is inaccurate. This statement was made in another CMNR report as shown. See suggested wording changes in AR 40-25REF.

Table 2-2. See suggested wording changes in AR 40-25REF. Also note that because of the inclusion of minimum requirements for potassium and chloride, the title for this table becomes incorrect and inappropriate. It is questionable if the values for potassium and chloride should even be included or presented as part of this table. The RDA table (Table II-1) includes a footnote indicating that desirable intakes of potassium may considerably exceed the minimum requirements (approx. 3,500 mg for adults) and there is further explanation/discussion in the text. The chloride value is not compatible with other statements regarding Na or NaCl.

Table 2-3. See suggested wording changes in AR 40-25REF.

NOTE: See Specific Statements earlier. This entire table needs accompanying text that indicates clearly how the values were derived.

Chapter 3 Nutrition Education

3-1. Introduction a-c. See suggested wording changes in AR 40-25REF.

3-2. Table 3-2 The CMNR suggests replacing the food guide pyramid (a copy of which we have added to C). Alternatively an additional new pyramid could be developed to become Table 3-3. In this new table, the suggested servings in the pyramid could be derived from values for energy in AR 40-25REV (2,250 kcal for women; 3,150 kcal for men).

    Line 605. We have added the text from the USDA and DHHS brochure (1990) that we assume you will include here in AR 40-25REF. The revision of the *Dietary Guidelines* is in progress (USDA, 1995), and new *Dietary Guidelines* are anticipated. These recommendations should also be considered in this section. In addition, there is a need to indicate the servings for higher caloric levels. As an example, these are the sample diets for a day at what are designated as Moderate and High calorie intakes in supporting documentation that accompanied the Food Pyramid. These would have to be modified further for inclusion in the revised text:

	MODERATE 2,200 Kcal	HIGH 3,150 Kcal
Bread Group Servings	9	11
Vegetable Group Servings	4	5
Fruit Group Servings	3	4
Milk Group Servings	2-3	2-3
Meat Group (ounces)	6	7
Total fat (g)	73	93
Total added sugars (tsp)	12	18

3-2b Sections (1) through (7) are direct extracts from the *Dietary Guidelines* (1990). No comments are warranted. The Army must consider the newly issued *Report of the Dietary Guidelines Advisory Committee on the Dietary Guidelines for Americans, 1995* (USDA, 1995) in revisions to this section.

APPENDIX A

References - A reference section needs to be added that includes all articles cited in the text in a consistent, scientific format.

Required and Recommended Reading See previous comments.

APPENDIX B Justification for Protein Recommendations

Note: The word "requirement" needs to be changed to "recommendation" throughout Appendix B. See suggested wording changes in AR 40-25REF.

g. Line 776: These values conflict with the values in **Table 2-1**: 3,600 for men; 2,500 for women. Which are the ones to be used?

Line 777: Table 2-1 values are 88 and 69 grams respectively. These are in conflict, which are correct?

APPENDIX C

Nutrient Density Index The CMNR was not provided with the necessary background material to review this Appendix. No detailed review or recommendations could therefore be provided here. There are several points worth noting about errors/confusion in Table C-1. Footnotes 1, 2 and 3 apply only to the values for the reduced calorie menu; thus the placement of the footnote numbers in the table is completely confusing. The values for minimum recommended allowance also are incorrect/confusing. The minimums are based on the minimums indicated in the RDAs for energy intakes <2,000 kcal, which are not the values listed in the footnotes.

GLOSSARY

Abbreviations. Add B Rations and T Rations and others from text.

Terms. See suggested wording changes in AR 40-25REF.

After definition for congregate feeding, please add definition for discretionary sodium such as, "Sodium which is added to foods by the cook or by the individual when food is eaten." As an alternative, the terms "discretionary" and "nondiscretionary" could be listed under the term sodium as separate items. In addition, the entire Terms section may need additional review to be sure that all terms are actually used in the text, for example, is cholecalciferol still cited in the text?

REFERENCES

AR 45-20. 1985. *See* U.S. Departments of the Army, the Navy, and the Air Force.

DHHS (U.S. Department of Health and Human Services). 1988. The Surgeon General's Report on Nutrition and Health. DHHS (PHS) Publ. No. 88-50210. Public Health Service, U.S. Department of Health and Human Services. Washington, D.C.: U.S. Government Printing Office.

IOM (Institute of Medicine). 1990. Nutrition During Pregnancy. Subcommittee on Nutritional Status and Weight Gain During Pregnancy, Subcommittee on Dietary Intake and Nutrient Supplements During Pregnancy, Committee on Nutritional Status During Pregnancy and Lactation, Food and Nutrition Board. Washington, D.C.: National Academy Press.

IOM. 1991a. Military Nutrition Initiatives. A Brief Report of the Committee on Military Nutrition Research, Food and Nutrition Board. February 25, 1991. Washington, D.C.: National Academy Press.

IOM. 1991b. Fluid Replacement and Heat Stress. Proceedings of a Workshop of the Committee on Military Nutrition Research, Food and Nutrition Board. Washington, D.C.: National Academy Press.

IOM. 1991c. Nutrition During Lactation. Subcommittee on Nutrition During Pregnancy, Committee on Nutritional Status During Pregnancy and Lactation, Food and Nutrition Board. Washington, D.C.: National Academy Press.

IOM. 1992a. Body Composition and Physical Performance, Applications for the Military Services. Committee on Military Nutrition Research, Food and Nutrition Board. Washington, D.C.: National Academy Press.

IOM. 1992b. Fluid Replacement and Heat Stress, 2nd printing. Committee on Military Nutrition Research, Food and Nutrition Board. Washington, D.C.: National Academy Press.

IOM. 1992c. Nutrition During Pregnancy and Lactation: An Implementation Guide. Subcommittee for a Clinical Application Guide, Committee on Nutritional Status During Pregnancy and Lactation, Food and Nutrition Board. Washington, D.C.: National Academy Press.

IOM. 1993. Nutritional Needs in Hot Environments, Applications for Military Personnel in Field Operations. Committee on Military Nutrition Research, Food and Nutrition Board. Washington, D.C.: National Academy Press.

IOM. 1994a. Fluid Replacement and Heat Stress, 3rd printing. Committee on Military Nutrition Research, Food and Nutrition Board. Washington, D.C.: National Academy Press.

IOM. 1994b. How Should the Recommended Dietary Allowances Be Revised? Food and Nutrition Board. Washington, D.C.: National Academy Press.

NRC (National Research Council). 1989a. Diet and Health: Implications for Reducing Chronic Disease Risk. Committee on Diet and Health, Food and Nutrition Board, Commission on Life Sciences. Washington, D.C.: National Academy Press.

NRC. 1989b. Recommended Dietary Allowances, 10th ed. Report of the Subcommittee on the Tenth Edition of the RDAs, Food and Nutrition Board, Commission on Life Sciences. Washington, D.C.: National Academy Press.

USDA (U.S. Department of Agriculture). 1995. Report of the Dietary Guidelines Advisory Committee on the Dietary Guidelines for Americans, 1995. Washington, D.C.: U.S. Government Printing Office.

USDA and DHHS (U.S. Department of Agriculture and U.S. Department of Health and Human Services). 1990. Dietary Guidelines for Americans, 3rd ed. Washington, D.C.: U.S. Government Printing Office.

U.S. Departments of the Army, the Navy, and the Air Force. 1985. Army Regulation 40-25/Naval Command Medical Instruction 10110.1/Air Force Regulation 160-95. "Nutrition Allowances, Standards, and Education." May 15. Washington, D.C.

Appendix E

Letter Report: Review of Issues Related to Iron Status in Women During U.S. Army Basic Combat Training

Submitted December 1995

FOOD AND NUTRITION BOARD
COMMITTEE ON MILITARY NUTRITION RESEARCH

(202) 334-1737
FAX (202) 334-2316

December 19, 1995

Brig. General R. Zajtchuk
Commanding General
U.S. Army Medical Research and Materiel
  Command (SGRD-ZA)
Fort Detrick
Frederick, MD 21702-5012

Dear General Zajtchuk:

At the specific request of Harris R. Lieberman, Ph.D., Chief, Military Nutrition Division, U.S. Army Research Institute of Environmental Medicine (USARIEM) and Grant Officer Representative of the U.S. Army Medical Research and Materiel Command (the Command) for Grant No. DAMD17-94-J-4046 to the National Academy of Sciences for support of the Food and Nutrition Board's (FNB) Committee on Military Nutrition Research (CMNR), members of the CMNR met in Washington, D.C. on November 13, 1995. The purpose of this meeting was to provide additional scientific guidance to the staff of the Military Nutrition Division in reviewing their recent research related to iron deficiency in military women during U.S. Army Basic Combat Training. The CMNR was requested to perform this review as part of its task to provide scientific support to USARIEM, which has the mission to perform military nutrition and related research.

Prior to the meeting, the CMNR reviewed (1) *Nutritional Assessment of Cadets at the U.S. Military Academy: Part 1. Anthropometric & Biochemical Measures* (Friedl et al., 1990); (2) *Nutritional Assessment of Cadets at the U.S. Military Academy: Part 2. Assessment of Nutritional Intake* (Klicka et al., 1993); (3) *Relationship between Iron Status and Physical Performance in Female Soldiers during U.S. Army Basic Combat Training* (Westphal et al., 1995); (4) *Health, Performance, and Nutrition Status of U.S. Army Women during Basic Combat Training* (Draft manuscript, K. A. Westphal, K. E. Friedl, M. A. Sharp, N. King, T. R. Kramer, K. L. Reynolds, and L. J. Marchitelli, U.S. Army Research Institute of Environmental Medicine, 1995); and (5) the recent FNB report, *Iron Deficiency Anemia* (IOM, 1993). These materials are

123

appended to the report with the materials presented to the CMNR for review at the meeting and a list of meeting participants.

The Committee on Military Nutrition Research's role at the meeting was to review the previously published Army technical reports and new material presented at the meeting. The Committee was asked to write a formal report that included responses to nine questions posed by Dr. Lieberman and MAJ Karl E. Friedl, Ph.D., and to evaluate, comment upon, and make specific recommendations regarding these studies and proposed research plans. Drs. John L. Beard and Sean Lynch served as special consultants to the CMNR for this project. These consultants participated in the meeting and the initial discussion with the Committee regarding this report. The report was written by the CMNR and represents the Committee's views concerning the issues.

This report has two parts. Part I is this letter that contains the conclusions and general recommendations of the CMNR. Part II includes the specific answers to the questions posed by the Army representatives.

This report of the CMNR has been reviewed in accordance with National Research Council (NRC) guidelines by a separate anonymous scientific review panel. This report is thus based on executive session discussions by the Committee and is a thoughtfully developed presentation incorporating the scientific opinion of the CMNR and the comments of the anonymous peer review panel of the NRC.

CONCLUSIONS AND RECOMMENDATIONS

The CMNR presents the following conclusions and recommendations to the U.S. Army Medical Research and Materiel Command regarding iron deficiency in military women during U.S. Army Basic Combat Training (BCT).

Conclusions

It is the view of the CMNR that iron status is an important issue for military women. From the preliminary data presented at this meeting, the potential for some compromise in physical performance has been demonstrated with low iron stores. Of equal military concern are the possible effects on cognitive performance that may result from impaired iron nutrition. Therefore, additional research should be conducted on the most susceptible groups of military women. It is important to determine whether the compromised iron status observed in women in BCT affects performance; therefore, initial studies should emphasize this issue, using an iron supplement that has the greatest potential for preventing or correcting decrements in iron status with appropriate nutrition counseling stressing the importance of taking such supplements, to help assure compliance with the study design. Following this determination, it then will be important to determine whether appropriate nutrition education methods can achieve similar results.

Since the stresses of military training are an approximation of the anticipated stresses of actual combat, it is important to collect and evaluate broadly all pertinent information from women involved in rigorous, physically stressful military training.

Any analysis of iron status must take into consideration the possible presence of any concurrent infectious or inflammatory processes, which are known to affect rapidly the results of clinical laboratory parameters used to measure iron status.

Recommendations

As a result of the review and discussion of related information, the CMNR recommends that:

• Intervention studies be conducted with women in BCT to identify cognitive and physical performance decrements that may be related to iron status.

• An evaluation of the most appropriate approaches to correcting deficits in iron status be made (i.e., nutrition education versus iron supplements).

• An analysis of existing data be conducted using models of iron deficiency previously recommended for the NHANES II and III studies.

• A screening program for military women be established to identify the extent of deficits in iron status and periods of greatest vulnerability, in order that remedial steps can be instituted where appropriate.

• Enlistment of any individual with iron deficiency anemia be delayed until this medically-reversible condition has been corrected.

Future Research Considerations

• Evaluate the effectiveness of dietary intervention using nutrition education in maintaining iron status.

• Evaluate the impact of dieting measures to meet weight standards on iron status and the potential for nutrition educational approaches to assist women in maintaining iron status when restricting calorie consumption.

• If a relationship between iron status and physical and cognitive performance is found, determine the measure of iron deficiency that best correlates with performance and the extent of iron deficiency that results in a compromised performance.

• In conjunction with monitoring iron status of military women, survey the impact of iron (and other macro- and micronutrient) status on immune function and the impact of iron status on the cardiovascular and pulmonary systems.

• If studies confirm instances of compromised iron status (in individuals who are free of active infections or inflammatory processes), evaluate various delivery systems to minimize or eliminate deficits in iron status such as:

  • a diet naturally high in iron (along with nutrition education), and
  • periodic nutritional supplements of iron (e.g., daily, weekly) (following a review of the dosage and effectiveness [as well as risk of complications such as gastrointestinal side-effects] as reported in the scientific literature).

• If such delivery systems prove to be ineffective, consider the evaluation of other interventions, such as:

  • iron delivered orally in a hydrodynamically balanced solution (Cook et al., 1990), and
  • the safety and effectiveness of oral heme iron.

The CMNR is pleased to provide this review as part of the Committee's continuing response to the U.S. Army Medical Research and Materiel Command. The Committee always welcomes comments and suggestions from you or your staff regarding how these reports can better serve the needs of the Army.

Sincerely,

Robert O. Nesheim, Ph.D.
Chairman, Committee on Military Nutrition Research

Attachments

cc: COL J. T. Hiatt
     MAJ K. E. Friedl
     F. W. Hagge
     H. R. Lieberman
     K. I. Shine
     K. Hein
     A. A. Yates
     S. J. Carlson

REFERENCES

Cook, J.D., M. Carriaga, S.G. Kahn, W. Schalch, and B.S. Skikne. 1990. Gastric delivery system for iron supplementation. Lancet 335:1136–1139.

Friedl, K.E., L.J. Marchitelli, D.E. Sherman, and R. Tulley. 1990. Nutritional assessment of cadets at the U.S. Military Academy: Part 1. Anthropometric & biochemical measures. Technical report T4-91. Natick, Mass.: U.S. Army Research Institute of Environmental Medicine.

IOM (Institute of Medicine). 1993. Iron Deficiency Anemia: Recommended Guidelines for the Prevention, Detection, and Management among U.S. Children and Women of Childbearing Age. A report of the Committee on the Prevention, Detection, and Management of Iron Deficiency Anemia Among U.S. Children and Women of Childbearing Age, Food and Nutrition Board. Washington, D.C.: National Academy Press.

Klicka, M.V., D.E. Sherman, N. King, K.E. Friedl, and E.W. Askew. 1993. Nutritional assessment of cadets at the U.S. Military Academy: Part 2. Assessment of Nutritional Intake. Technical report T94-1. Natick, Mass.: U.S. Army Research Institute of Environmental Medicine.

Westphal, K.A., L.J. Marchitelli, K.E. Friedl, and M.A. Sharp. 1995. Relationship between iron status and physical performance in female soldiers during U.S. Army Basic Combat Training [abstract]. Fed. Am. Soc. Exp. Biol. J. 9(3):A361.

Part II

ANSWERS TO THE NINE SPECIFIC QUESTIONS PRESENTED TO THE CMNR BY THE ARMY REPRESENTATIVES

The answers to the nine specific questions posed to the CMNR are:

1. Do the data from recent research studies indicate that there is a problem related to iron deficiency in Army women in U.S. Army Basic Combat Training (BCT)?

Two recent military studies offer evidence that a significant number of female trainees has suboptimal iron stores. In one, a significant fraction of women cadets at the U.S. Military Academy (USMA) was observed to have below normal values of one or more markers of iron status (hematocrit [Hct], hemoglobin [Hgb], serum ferritin, iron saturation, serum iron, and total iron-binding capacity). In the other study conducted at Fort Jackson, new army recruits entered BCT with below normal serum ferritin values, which were reduced even further during the course of 8 weeks of BCT. Such information indicates suboptimal iron status, though other indices did not change (notably Hct and Hgb). It is not known whether the subjects' physical or cognitive performance was impaired as a result of this deficiency in body iron stores, though data in the literature have linked diminished iron status to possible impairment of these functions. The USMA results suggest a high incidence of chronically impaired iron stores. Due to disparity in the definitions of iron status, it is not yet possible to directly compare the BCT results, which indicated rapid depletion of iron stores under conditions of demanding physical activity, with those of the USMA study, which involved female cadets.

2. Do the data indicate that the incidence of iron deficiency or low iron stores among military women is different from what exists in women with the same demographic characteristics in the civilian population?

Given available data, it seems clear that a sizable fraction of the population of both military and civilian women exhibit a significant degree of diminished iron storage, but it is not yet possible, due to disparity in the definitions of iron status, to compare directly the relative degrees of compromised iron status. Profiles of iron status of military women entering BCT were similar to those of civilian women with comparable demographic characteristics, as presented in preliminary form at the meeting (NHANES III, Personal communication, A. C. Looker, National Center for Health Statistics, 1995).

The NHANES III defined iron deficiency according to two separate models or sets of criteria. The "Ferritin" model defines iron deficiency as abnormal levels of two or more of the following: serum ferritin concentration, percent transferrin saturation (TS), and red blood cell (RBC) protoporphyrin concentration. The Mean Cell Volume (MCV) model defines iron deficiency as abnormal levels of two or more of the following: MCV, TS, and RBC protoporphyrin. For women ages 20 to 49, the cutoff levels (as determined by the 2.5th percentile values) were: serum ferritin concentration less than 12 ng/ml, TS less than 15 percent, RBC protoporphyrin concentration greater than 70 µg/dL, and MCV less than 85 fl.

Iron deficiency anemia was defined as a Hgb concentration less than 118 g/L accompanied by two or more of the Ferritin or MCV model criteria for iron deficiency. According to data from Phase I of NHANES III (Personal communication, A. C. Looker, National Center for Health Statistics, 1995; Dallman et al., in press), the prevalence of iron deficiency among non-African American women ages 20 to 49 was 9 to 10 percent (comparable data for African-American women are not yet available), whereas the prevalence of iron deficiency anemia was 3 to 4 percent among non-African American women ages 20 to 49. In comparison, a followup survey of iron status among female Army enlisted women, average age 21 years (data not available by ethnic group) at the beginning of BCT utilized a serum ferritin concentration of less than 12 ng/ml as the criterion for iron deficiency and a combination of low serum ferritin and Hgb of less than 120 g/L as the criteria for iron deficiency anemia (thus, these definitions would include some women who would be excluded using NHANES criteria). Seventeen percent of new female recruits surveyed fit these criteria for iron deficiency, while 8 percent could be classified as having iron deficiency anemia.

A survey of a similar population at the end of BCT showed that, by that time, 33 percent were iron deficient, and 26 percent were anemic (the prevalence of iron deficiency with and without anemia did not differ significantly between African American and non-African American recruits) (Personal communication, LTC A. Cline, U.S. Army Research Institute of Environmental Medicine, 1995).

Studies in civilian women athletes show reductions in iron stores with physical training (Lyle et al., 1992), similar to those observed in women recruits undergoing BCT. In general, however, military women are more vulnerable than civilian women to developing depleted iron stores due to the demands placed on them for vigorous physical activity. A careful comparison has not yet been made, and it is thus not possible to conclude whether the military population of women differs from the civilian population regarding iron status. Regardless, compromised iron status should be of great concern to the Army because of the need to maintain military personnel in a high state of physical and mental readiness.

3. In terms of military readiness, would military women benefit from a nutritional intervention?

Military readiness can be compromised by severely depleted iron stores. At present, the degree of iron depletion necessary to cause meaningful decrements in physical and cognitive performance is unknown. Hence, it is not possible to conclude that an intervention would improve military readiness until the degree of decrement is correlated with performance. Some available data suggest that physical performance is impaired by subnormal iron status (Westphal et al., 1995), but the literature is not conclusive regarding the level of suboptimal stores necessary for impairment (Edgerton et al., 1979; Gardner et al., 1977).

Too few data exist to evaluate whether cognitive performance in military women is affected by poor iron status. Iron deficiency anemia has been associated with lowered scores on tests of discrimination learning in infants and children, suggestive of disturbances in attentional processes. To date, most studies have failed to document significant relationships between iron deficiency and cognitive changes in the absence of anemia (Pollitt et al., 1986) but sufficient controversy remains to merit further research.

The negative impact of significant physical stress on iron status is well documented (Haymes and Lamanca, 1989). With the demonstrated reduction in iron status during BCT, it is possible that iron status might be further diminished during combat duty. Since no data are currently available to evaluate this possibility, this issue demands further investigation. In particular, the impact on iron status of physical exercise of the intensity experienced during BCT and combat needs to be evaluated.

It is important that measures to correct low iron status be accomplished on an individual basis. Iron fortification levels in cereal grain products have been designed to meet the needs of most individuals without causing harm associated with too much iron intake. As reviewed by the IOM (1993), excess iron stores have been linked, at least theoretically, to an increased incidence of ischemic heart disease, as well as several types of cancers and neurological disorders. There is evidence that excess dietary iron may also interfere with absorption of dietary zinc (Zn) and copper (Cu) and iron supplementation may cause gastrointestinal side-effects. For these reasons, blanket iron supplementation of all military women is not prudent.

4. Are there additional medical considerations related to iron status in military women that need to be addressed?

Yes. Examples include reproductive health, function of the immune, cardiovascular and pulmonary systems, and the greater consequences of blood loss, such as through blood donation or wounds. In most studies, these potential problems have not been thoroughly investigated.

5. Should there be periodic screening of military women for anemia or iron deficiency?

Yes. Annual screening (detection) should evaluate iron status and identify both iron deficiency and iron deficiency anemia (by including an initial measurement of serum ferritin). Those identified with low serum ferritin values should be further evaluated by other criteria such as Hgb, Hct, RBC protoporphyrin, and possibly circulating transferrin receptors. Infectious diseases and inflammatory processes are known to alter the results of laboratory indicators of iron nutrition, and therefore the presence of any such medical problem must be identified and noted at the time of screening. Evaluation of the status of other nutrients that may result in anemias, such as vitamin B_6, vitamin B_{12}, and folate should be performed on an annual basis as well.

Screening should be done in the following manner:

a) At the time of initial entry into service.

Those persons with a clear-cut diagnosis of iron deficiency anemia (the exact criteria to confirm this diagnosis must be defined for this military purpose, including any possible racial differences) should have their enlistment deferred until this correctable medical condition can be reversed by proper therapy. Since 53 percent of active duty Army women are classified as belonging to a minority group (44 percent of Army women are African American) (IOM, 1995), racial differences in diagnostic criteria for iron deficiency anemia need to be considered for accession and treatment.

b) Upon completion of BCT.

Those individuals with iron deficiency or iron deficiency anemia should receive appropriate medical treatment, and be monitored until laboratory results show a return to normal values. Current recommendations for treatment include a daily 6-week course of high dose supplemental iron with nutritional counseling, followed by monitoring of Hgb and either continuation of the high dose or adjustment to a maintenance level (LSRO, 1991).

c) In women on active military duty, at the time of their required annual Pap Smear exam (IOM, 1995).

Those individuals with iron deficiency or iron deficiency anemia should receive appropriate medical treatment.

d) At the time of any initial prenatal visit, and throughout any pregnancy, as previously recommended (IOM, 1993).

Those women with laboratory evidence of iron deficiency or iron deficiency anemia should receive appropriate medical treatment.

e) At the time of a woman's 4–6 week post-partum visit.

Those with iron deficiency or iron deficiency anemia should receive appropriate medical treatment.

f) Women who are identified clinically as being at high risk for developing iron deficiency should be screened at more frequent, medically-defined intervals.

g) Results from all screening studies related to iron nutrition should be entered into an individual's medical records and assessed clinically on a longitudinal basis.

6. In military personnel with low iron stores as well as anemia, is there an impairment of military readiness that is gender specific?

Iron deficiency anemia can be expected to have adverse effects on the military performance of both men and women, depending in part upon its severity. Performance deficits in both men and women due to compromised iron status have been demonstrated most clearly during exercise of prolonged duration, such as long distance running (Newhouse and Clement, 1988). Iron deficiency anemia may also have an adverse impact upon recovery from serious wounds or injuries, especially those that involve large blood loss.

Mild iron deficiency without anemia has been shown to produce decrements in physical performance in rats (Zinker et al., 1993); however, comparable experiments have not been carried out in humans. Research in this area should be expanded.

It is clear that women experience a far greater variability than men in the status of their iron stores. This problem is partially due to variable menstrual blood losses, parity, pregnancy, and any terminations of pregnancy. In addition, dietary intake of iron (and energy) tends to be lower in women than in men. Self-imposed dieting is more prevalent among women (Klicka et al., 1993) and adds to the risk for lowered iron stores. BCT also impacts the iron stores of women to a greater degree than those of men (Moore et al., 1993). Voluntary blood donation has a greater impact on the iron status of women than it does on men (LSRO, 1991).

Iron nutrition may be an issue in achieving gender-neutral job standards for military occupational specialties (MOS's).

7. Are there additional analyses that should be conducted with the data in Friedl et al., 1990 ; Klicka et al., 1993; Westphal et al., 1995; or Westphal et al. [draft manuscript], 1995 on iron status issues in women in BCT? For future studies, are there additional specific analyses that should be considered?

In evaluating the data presented in Army technical reports (Friedl et al., 1990; Klicka et al., 1993; Westphal et al., 1995; Westphal et al. [draft manuscript], 1995) and in future studies, consideration should be given to using NHANES II and III models for identifying iron deficiency and iron deficiency anemia. Two such models which are established are the Ferritin model and the MCV model. The ferritin model includes the use of data on serum ferritin, the percent TS, and RBC protoporphyrin levels. The MCV model uses the MCV, percent TS, and RBC protoporphyrin values. The rationale for using these models is described in the report, *Summary of a Report on Assessment of the Iron Nutritional Status of the United States Population* (Expert Scientific Group, 1985). In studies where a sufficient number of observations are available, consideration might also be given to using an analysis of the iron storage status of the whole population based on the model developed by Cook and colleagues (1986).

The inclusion of a new assay for detecting a deficiency of iron stores (the circulating transferrin receptor concentration) should also be considered. The concentration of this specific protein appears to be a direct measure of tissue iron demand and has the particular advantage of not being affected by infections. Concurrent infections reduce the reliability of measures of ferritin, TS, and erythrocyte protoporphyrin as indicators of iron deficiency (Cook et al., 1993; Flowers et al., 1989; Skikne et al., 1990). Therefore, additional analyses must consider the presence of coexisting problems of infection and inflammation.

With the data from the completed studies, analyses should be extended where possible and appropriate to include the impact of ethnic and lifestyle factors, such as smoking and alcohol consumption. Future studies should also consider the impact of aspirin and other non-steroidal, anti-inflammatory drugs on gastric blood loss.

8. What are the CMNR recommendations regarding the proposed intervention study?

In the proposed intervention study, if the primary objective is to determine the effect of compromised iron status on physical and cognitive performance, then the CMNR recommends consideration that a prospective intervention trial using iron supplements be conducted initially. If this study indicates clear positive effects on performance, then a subsequent study could be designed to evaluate nutrition education (i.e., dietary intervention without supplementation) as an alternative method for increasing iron intake. For the intervention trial, the following design changes are recommended:

Objectives:
    a) to determine whether iron deficiency and/or iron deficiency anemia affects selected military performance measures in participating subjects;
    b) to determine whether correction of iron deficiency will improve selected military performance measures;
    c) to determine whether a 60 mg or smaller iron supplement (dose to depend on a thorough review of iron supplementation research) will correct any observed iron deficiencies in participating subjects; and
    d) to determine whether participating subjects will tolerate a 60 mg daily elemental iron supplement.

Type of Study:
    Prospective intervention trial with placebo controls.

Study Population:
    If at all possible, the desired study population should be BCT personnel. Such trainees have been shown to be at greatest risk for developing iron deficiency or iron deficiency anemia during training. In addition, the use of this population would provide data comparable to those generated in previous Army studies.
    The use of advanced individual training (AIT) personnel is less desirable because they have just been subjected to 8 weeks of BCT. Studies have demonstrated that measures of iron status tend to stabilize by 12 weeks, and physiological adaptation or compensatory reaction may take place (Blum et al., 1986; Rajaram et al., 1991). Moreover, no complete studies have been done previously in AIT personnel.

Design of Study:
    A 2 x 2 randomized, ethnically balanced block factorial design of 8-week duration in BCT volunteers is recommended, with a stratified assignment of subjects to inadequate iron stores (IIS) and adequate iron stores (AIS) groups. The CMNR assumes that no person who is classified with iron deficiency anemia will be included (as discussed in the response to Question 5). Within each stratum subjects will be randomized to placebo versus intervention groups. Intervention will consist of a daily supplement containing 60 mg or less of elemental iron in the form of ferrous sulfate tablets. Ideally, iron tablets should be taken in the fasting state with a glass of orange juice. Counseling on this point and on the importance of adherence is essential. Compliance must be enforced and monitored.
    Power analysis should be performed to determine the sample size required to demonstrate statistically significant effects.

Group hematology:

IIS:	Hgb	≤	12 g/dL
	Ferritin	<	20 ug/L
	TS	≤	16 %
AIS:	Hgb	≥	12 g/dL
	Ferritin	>	20 ug/L
	TS	>	16 %

What is Measured:

a) Hematologic responses;

b) cognitive and physical performance variables should be emphasized, such as

i) endurance performance (e.g., 2 mile run) in the physical tests and

ii) cognitive tests, particularly those involving attention;

c) full recording of infectious illnesses and inflammatory conditions incurred during the study; plus useful laboratory markers such as RBC Sedimentation Rates, G reactive protein, and plasma haptoglobin; and

d) side effects,

i) especially gastrointestinal and

ii) if a 60 mg daily iron supplement is used, zinc and copper status should be monitored since there is some evidence to suggest that excess iron supplementation may interfere with the absorption of dietary zinc and copper (IOM 1993).

Depending on the results of this intervention, a subsequent intervention should be conducted to evaluate the efficacy of a nutritional education program in correcting iron deficiency. Design of such a program should be based in part on a careful evaluation of dietary habits of subjects in earlier studies, particularly with respect to iron intake, restricted eating and food preferences.

9. Emphasis of the meeting on November 13, 1995 was on data collected during BCT, should there be additional research with military women dealing with iron status in military women in general?

Yes. Data should be collected to investigate the iron status of career military women, as recommended in the answer to Question 5 regarding screening.

REFERENCES

Blum, S.M., A.R. Sherman, and R.A. Boileau. 1986. The effects of fitness-type exercise on iron status in adult women. Am. J. Clin. Nutr. 43:456–463.

Cook, J.D., B.S. Skikne, S.R. Lynch, and M.E. Reusser. 1986. Estimates of iron sufficiency in the U.S. population. Blood 68:726–731.

Cook, J.D., M. Carriaga, S.G. Kahn, W. Schalch, and B.S. Skikne. 1990. Gastric delivery system for iron supplementation. Lancet 335:1136–1139.

Cook, J.D., B.S. Skikne, and R.D. Baynes. 1993. Serum transferrin receptor. Annu. Rev. Med. 44:63–74.

Dallman, P., A. C. Looker, C.L. Johnson, and M. Carroll. In Press. Influence of age on laboratory criteria for the diagnosis of iron deficiency anemia and iron deficiency in infants and children. In Proceedings of Symposium on Iron Nutrition in Health and Disease, L. Halberg, ed. London: John Lubbey and Company.

Edgerton, V.R., G.W. Gardner, Y. Ohira, K.A. Gunawardina, and B. Senewiratne. 1979. Iron-deficiency anemia and its effect on worker productivity and activity patterns. Br. Med. J. 2:1546–1549.

Expert Scientific Working Group of the Life Sciences Research Office, FASEB. 1988. Summary of a report on assessment of the iron nutritional status of the United States population. Am. J. Clin. Nutr. 42:1318–1330.

Flowers, C.H., B.S. Skikne, A.M. Covell, and J.D. Cook. 1989. The clinical measurement of serum transferrin receptor. J. Lab. Clin. Med. 114:368–377.

Friedl, K.E., L.J. Marchitelli, D.E. Sherman, and R. Tulley. 1990. Nutritional assessment of cadets at the U.S. Military Academy: Part 1. Anthropometric & biochemical measures. Technical report T4-91. Natick, Mass.: U.S. Army Research Institute of Environmental Medicine.

Gardner, G.W., V.R. Edgerton, B. Senewiratne, R.J. Barnard, and Y. Ohira. 1977. Physical work capacity and metabolic stress in subjects with iron deficiency anemia. Am. J. Clin. Nutr. 30:910–917.

Haymes, E.M., and J.J. Lamanca. 1989. Iron loss in runners during exercise: Implications and recommendations. Sports Medicine 7:277–285.

IOM (Institute of Medicine). 1993. Iron Deficiency Anemia: Recommended Guidelines for the Prevention, Detection, and Management among U.S. Children and Women of Childbearing Age. A report of the Committee on the Prevention, Detection, and Management of Iron Deficiency Anemia Among U.S. Children and Women of Childbearing Age, Food and Nutrition Board. Washington, D.C.: National Academy Press.

IOM. 1995. Recommendations for Research on the Health of Military Women. A report of the Committee on Defense Women's Health Research. Washington, D.C.: National Academy Press.

Klicka, M.V., D.E. Sherman, N. King, K.E. Friedl, and E.W. Askew. 1993. Nutritional assessment of cadets at the U.S. Military Academy: Part 2. Assessment of nutritional intake. Technical report T94-1. Natick, Mass.: U.S. Army Research Institute of Environmental Medicine.

LSRO (Life Sciences Research Office). 1991. Guidelines for the Assessment and Management of Iron Deficiency in Women of Childbearing Age. Prepared for Center for Food Safety and Applied Nutrition, Food and Drug Administration, U.S. Department of Health and Human Services. Bethesda, Md.: Life Sciences Research Office, Federation of American Societies for Experimental Biology.

Lyle, R.M., C.M. Weaver, D.A. Sedlock, S. Rajaram, B. Martin, and C.L. Melby. 1992. Iron status in exercising women: The effect of oral iron therapy vs. increased consumption of muscle foods. Am. J. Clin. Nutr. 56a:1049–1055.

Moore, R.J., K.E. Friedl, R.T. Tulley, and E.W. Askew. 1993. Maintenance of iron status in healthy men during an extended period of stress and physical activity. Am. J. Clin. Nutr. 58:923–927.

Newhouse, I.J., and D.B. Clement. 1988. Iron status in athletes. Sports Med. 5:337–352.

Pollitt, E., C. Saco-Pollitt, R.L. Leibel, and F.E. Viteri. 1986. Iron deficiency and behavioral development in infants and preschool children. Am. J. Clin. Nutr. 43:555–565.

Rajaram, S., C.M. Weaver, R.M. Lyle, D.A. Sedlock, and C.L. Melby. 1991. Effect of oral iron therapy vs. increased consumption of muscle foods on iron status in exercising women [abstract]. Fed. Am. Soc. Exp. Biol. J. 5:A1656.

Skikne, B.S., C.H. Flowers, and J.D. Cook. 1990. Serum transferrin receptor: A quantitative measure of tissue iron deficiency. Blood 75:1870–1876.

Westphal, K.A., L.J. Marchitelli, K.E. Friedl, and M.A. Sharp. 1995. Relationship between iron status and physical performance in female soldiers during U.S. Army Basic Combat Training [abstract]. Fed. Am. Soc. Exp. Biol. J. 9(3):A361.

Zinker, B.A., P.R. Dallman, and G.A. Brooks. 1993. Augmented glucoregulatory hormone concentrations during exhausting exercise in mildly iron-deficient rats. Am. J. Physiol. 265(4 Pt 2):R863–871.

**A Review of Issues Related to Iron Status in Women
during U.S. Army Basic Combat Training**

November 13–14, 1995
Foundry Building Room 2004
1055 Thomas Jefferson Street, N.W.
Washington, D.C. 20007
(202) 334-1911

PARTICIPANTS

November 13, 1995
  Presentation Session, 9:00 a.m.–1:00 p.m.
  Closed Discussion Session, 1:00 p.m.–5:00 p.m.
November 14, 1995
  Executive Session, 8:30 a.m.–12:00 p.m.

Committee Members
(All sessions except where noted)
Robert O. Nesheim, Ph.D. *(Chair)*
Salinas, CA

William R. Beisel, M.D.
The Johns Hopkins School of
  Hygiene and Public Health
Baltimore, MD

Gail E. Butterfield, Ph.D.
(available by fax to review report)
Palo Alto Veterans Administration
  Medical Center, and
Program in Human Biology,
  Stanford University
Palo Alto, CA

John D. Fernstrom, Ph.D.
University of Pittsburgh School of
  Medicine
Western Psychiatric Institute and
  Clinic
Pittsburgh, PA

G. Richard Jansen, Ph.D.
Department of Food Science and
  Human Nutrition
Colorado State University
Fort Collins, CO

Robin B. Kanarek, Ph.D.
(available by fax to review report)
Department of Psychology
Tufts University
Medford, MA

Orville A. Levander, Ph.D.
Nutrient Requirements and
  Functions Laboratory
USDA, ARS/BHNRC
Beltsville, MD

Gilbert A. Leveille, Ph.D.
(available by fax to review report)
Research and Technical Services
Nabisco Foods Group
East Hanover, NJ

John E. Vanderveen, Ph.D.
(Presentation and Executive Sessions)
Food and Drug Administration
Washington, DC

Douglas W. Wilmore, M.D.
(available by fax to review report)
Department of Surgery
Brigham and Women's Hospital
Boston, MA

Johanna T. Dwyer
(Presentation and Closed Discussion Sessions)
Frances Stern Nutrition Center and
    Department of Medicine
Tufts Medical School and New
    England Medical Center
Boston, MA

*Special Consultants
(Presentation and Closed Discussion sessions except where noted)*
John L. Beard, Ph.D.
Department of Nutrition
The Pennsylvania State University
University Park, PA

James D. Cook, M.D., M.Sc.
(did not attend; did not receive airline ticket)
Division of Hematology
University of Kansas Medical
    Center
Kansas City, KS

Sean Lynch, M.D.
Hematology and Oncology,
    Veterans Administration Medical
    Center
Eastern Virginia Medical School
Hampton, VA

Elaine R. Monsen, Ph.D.
(available by fax to review report)
Department of Nutritional Sciences
University of Washington
Seattle, WA

*Military Representatives
(Presentation session only)*
LTC Alana Cline
Military Nutrition Division
Occupational Health &
    Performance Directorate
U.S. Army Research Institute of
    Environmental Medicine
Natick, MA

MAJ Karl E. Friedl, Ph.D.
U.S. Army Medical Research and
    Materiel Command
Fort Detrick
Frederick, MD

LTC Dale Hill
Army Surgeon General's Office
Falls Church, VA

Harris R. Lieberman, Ph.D.
Military Nutrition Division
U.S. Army Research Institute of
    Environmental Medicine
Natick, MA

Speaker
(Presentation session only)
Anne Looker, Ph.D., R.D.
Chief of Nutrition Statistics Branch
National Center for Health Statistics
  tics
Hyattsville, MD

Staff
(All sessions)
Bernadette M. Marriott, Ph.D.
Sydne J. Carlson, Ph.D.
Allison A. Yates, Ph.D., R.D.
Susan M. Knasiak

Appendix F

Conclusions and Recommendations from the Workshop Report Nutritional Needs in Cold and in High-Altitude Environments

Submitted March 1996

Conclusions and Recommendations

As stated in Chapter 1, the Committee on Military Nutrition Research (CMNR) was asked to respond to 15 specific questions that address factors affecting nutrient requirements and food intake for work in cold and in high-altitude environments. The committee's responses to these questions appear below.

ANSWERS TO QUESTIONS POSED BY THE ARMY

Performance

1. What is the effect of cold or altitude exposure on muscle strength and endurance?

Cold and high-altitude exposure affects muscle strength and endurance through changes in cardiac output and oxygen uptake. Very cold environments that lower body temperature by more than 0.9°F (0.5°C) may limit maximal cardiac output and result in reduced maximum oxygen uptake. Because moderately cold environments lower muscle temperature, endurance of moderate physical activity actually can be theoretically increased if body core temperature can be maintained. There are conflicting data on the effects of cold exposure on muscle strength, and more research is needed to determine this relationship.

High altitudes can also affect physical performance because they decrease maximum oxygen uptake by approximately 10 percent for every 3,280 ft (1,000 m) increase in altitude. Endurance is also significantly reduced at high altitudes (see Chapter 1 in this volume). While acclimatization to high altitudes does not improve maximum oxygen capacity, endurance does improve (often as much as 50 percent or more) (see Chapter 1 in this volume).

2. Can diet influence these changes?

Maintenance of muscle structure and function over the long term depends on muscle strength and exercise. Muscle strength and endurance are influenced by diet through maintenance of muscle mass and the availability of appropriate substrates for muscle activity. Provision of adequate dietary energy under circumstances of either cold or high-altitude exposure will maximize the possibility of maintenance of muscle mass, and thus muscle strength. Conversely, inadequate energy intake will result in loss of muscle tissue with a concomitant decrease in strength and endurance.

Macronutrient composition of dietary intake may influence this process. In the cold or at high altitudes, protein requirements are not elevated above the needs of the individual at ambient temperature or at sea level performing the same level of activity. Nevertheless, dietary protein should be adequate to maintain the muscle mass that supports the strenuous physical activity performed. Fat as a source of energy is well tolerated in the cold, but provision of adequate carbohydrate is important because it is the major fuel needed for shivering, an important method for maintaining body temperature, and thus indirectly affects endurance. At high altitudes, carbohydrate becomes the predominant fuel at rest and during exercise. Failure to supply sufficient energy as carbohydrate (at least 400 g/d) at high altitudes can result in loss of muscle mass and decreased endurance.

3. How does cold or altitude exposure influence appetite?

The term appetite in this context is defined as a desire for food or drink. The traditional wisdom has been that cold climatic conditions lead to an increase in appetite. The evidence for this conclusion is derived from changes in body weight, self-scored questionnaires, and food intake records in cold environments at sea level. However, the reported increase in appetite is also associated with changes in other aspects of the subjects' environment such as altered activity levels, isolation, reduced social interaction, and modifications in diet. Nonetheless, it does appear that food intake is generally increased with cold exposure.

With ascent to altitudes above 10,000 to 12,000 ft (3,048 to 3,658 m), food consumption is reduced regardless of temperature. Body weight loss is common among subjects during the first few weeks at high altitudes, and such weight loss can be avoided only with successful efforts to consume food.

Although some studies have reported weight gain in cold environments, other investigations have found that soldiers operating in cold climates may not consume military rations in amounts adequate to meet energy expenditure. Reports from field training exercises have shown decreased intake of energy relative to need in both cold and high-altitude environments. The factors that influence ration consumption discussed in the CMNR's report on *Not Eating*

Enough (IOM, 1995) may be even more significant for operations in the cold and in high altitudes. Encouragement of food discipline through a field feeding doctrine (IOM, 1995) would help soldiers maintain an appropriate level of food intake. With adaptation to altitude, appetite increases but generally food intake is insufficient to regain lost weight or even to maintain the lower weight.

Health and Medical Aspects

4. Is there concern for increased cardiovascular risk when a high fat diet is consumed for intermittent (7- to 14-d) time periods in the cold?

Although this question was not addressed specifically by any participant in the workshop, all available evidence indicates that there should be no concern with higher fat diets for these short periods of time. A major nutritional problem during military operations in the cold is meeting the added requirements for water and food to prevent both dehydration and weight loss. King et al. (1993) reported that in arctic field tests, the Army's 18-Man Arctic Tray Pack Ration Module[1] (29 percent of calories from fat), in combination with either a wet-pack (Meal, Ready-to-Eat[1] [MRE, 36 percent of calories from fat]) or a dehydrated (Long-Range Patrol, Improved[1] [LRP I, 35 percent of calories from fat]) individual ration, met the full daily nutritional recommendations for protein and micronutrients. However, energy needs were not met, and soldiers consistently lost body weight.

The easiest way for military feeding systems to provide for increased caloric needs during cold-weather operations is to include additional dietary fats. Such an increase in dietary fat is also most expedient, logistically. However, some tested supplements, containing only a modestly higher fat content, did not result in sufficient energy intake to prevent weight loss (Edwards and Roberts, 1991). Cold-weather operations probably require a total energy intake ranging from 45 to 62 kcal/kg body weight/d, but earlier military studies in the Arctic suggested that 4,000 kcal/d or less were actually being consumed (LeBlanc, 1957). Current projections for energy needs in arctic conditions focus on 58 kcal/kg body weight/d (see Chapter 1 in this volume).

Controversial questions about the relationships between dietary intakes of fat and cholesterol and the pathogenesis of atherosclerosis, strokes, and coronary heart disease have fueled important clinical research studies for several decades. Although recent estimations indicate that the average total fat intake in the United States has declined to 34 percent of total calories (CDC; 1994), the most recent review of national dietary guidelines recommends that an individual consume no more than 30 percent, with an increased intake of complex carbohydrates to provide total energy needs (USDA, 1995). Increased consumption of

---

[1] See Table 1-3 in Chapter 1 for total nutrient composition.

fruits and vegetables, which would increase the intake of complex carbohydrates, is also recommended.

However, these recommendations for the diet of the general population may not be appropriate for the military and logistical requirements for conducting either short- or long-term field operations in arctic climates. Fresh fruits and vegetables would be impossible to supply. Although diets supplying 58 kcal/kg body weight/d can be formulated with only 30 percent fat, they may prove operationally difficult to provide and the CMNR believes that this guideline is too restrictive for military operational rations. Diets containing more of the high density fat fuels may become an operational necessity. In addition, as pointed out by Edwards et al. (1992), the choice of ration must consider water availability, size and volume of load, resupply schedule, logistics, and the task at hand. Although a higher fat diet is clearly not a nutritional necessity in the Arctic, it may prove to be a logistical need.

From a metabolic point of view, it is probable that the additional fat calories will be metabolized promptly, to satisfy immediate energy needs, rather than being stored in body fat depots. If extra dietary fat is consumed primarily to meet high daily energy requirements and to prevent weight loss during military operations in cold climates, it will not necessarily have important long-term consequences.

Current national dietary recommendations have been in effect for only a few years, and there is no available research evidence to suggest that a temporary deviation from a low fat diet, eaten in order to meet unusually high energy demands, would have a long-term effect on slowly developing cardiovascular pathology.

If this question is viewed from a risk/benefit perspective, the short-term risks to a soldier who must participate in a dangerous military operation in arctic cold are high, and nutritional assistance must be given to help the soldier function at an optimal level. Clearly, inadequate energy intakes and progressive weight losses are not desirable. The immediate benefits of an adequate energy intake far outweigh the possibility that a short-term intake of extra fat calories (eaten to meet the energy demands of cold, arctic climates) might contribute to deleterious health effects several decades later.

5. What nutrients prevent or lessen the symptoms of acute altitude exposure?

Two nutrients have the reputation of being protective against acute mountain sickness (AMS): water and carbohydrate. Because acute altitude exposure is accompanied by diuresis in most individuals, replacement of water lost through diuresis has been reputed to be important in minimizing the symptoms of mountain sickness. Scientific data on this question are minimal. More careful studies have been done on the effect of carbohydrate feeding during acute exposure to altitude, and the general consensus from those studies is that carbohydrate is of benefit in minimizing the symptoms of acute exposure (Consolazio et al., 1969). Because carbohydrate is the primary metabolic fuel at rest and during exercise (Brooks et al., 1991; Roberts et al., in press a, b), and because it provides slightly more energy for the oxygen consumed than does fat (Kleiber, 1961), provision of ample amounts of this macronutrient could be expected to overcome the 500 kcal/d deficit created by exposure to hypobaric hypoxia, maintain body glycogen stores, and assist in the maintenance of muscle mass.

6. Is free radical formation a concern for prolonged (10- to 30-d) military operations at 10,000–15,000 ft (3,048–4,572 m) elevation?

Free radical formation, the consequence of oxidative stress, might be expected to increase in cold or in high altitude environments, due to (1) the elevation in metabolic rate that results from an increased energy expenditure; (2) the stress of hypoxia at altitude; and (3) the increased exposure to ultraviolet radiation at altitude or on snow-covered ground. As recently reviewed by Askew (1995), some limited evidence does suggest an increase in oxidative stress in high altitude environments. During a 6-wk polar expedition, an increase in production of malonaldehyde, a product of lipid peroxidation believed to be a marker for oxidative stress, was measured in erythrocytes and plasma, followed by decreased blood concentrations of vitamin E (Panin et al., 1992 as reported by Askew, 1995). Simon-Schnass (see Chapter 21 in this volume) also reported increased exhalation of pentane, another marker for oxidative stress, with prolonged stays at high altitudes. Further research is needed to assess the physiological significance of such markers in terms of actual oxidative tissue damage as well as the potential long-term consequence of such damage, and the likelihood for significant oxidative damage during the timeframe of typical military deployments to high-altitude areas. Thus, there appears to be a potential for increased oxidative stress at high altitudes. However, the possible long-term consequences as well as the extent to which any ensuing damage would be decreased or prevented by providing additional antioxidant nutrients are not known at this time, but this is an important area for future research.

Thermoregulation and Acclimatization

7. Is cold/altitude acclimatization facilitated by prior nutritional status or supplemental nutrients?

There are few data on this topic. Prior nutritional status may affect acclimatization to cold/altitude in that an individual in poor nutritional status may have difficulty in adapting. Nutrients of particular concern would be iron, because of its relationship to hemoglobin and hemoglobin synthesis, and vitamin E, because of its relationship to oxidative stress.

In addition to prior nutritional status, the body composition, recent losses of body weight or lean body mass, and recent health and training history of individual soldiers should be considered prior to their participation in missions or training in cold and in high-altitude environments. In particular, the extreme losses of lean body mass described for some individuals who participated in U.S. Army Ranger Training would need to be regained prior to working in environmental extremes.

8. What nutrients influence thermoregulation?

Thermoregulation involves cardiovascular measures to reduce heat loss (nonshivering thermogenesis), an increase in metabolic heat production through shivering and an increase in voluntary muscular activity.

In short term studies, shivering thermogenesis, like voluntary muscular activity, has been found to be fueled by carbohydrate and, to a lesser extent, fat. There is no evidence for a role for protein in shivering thermogenesis at this time; however, more research is needed to establish whether a specific proportion of nutrients has any advantage in maintaining thermoregulation under field conditions.

Thiamin, niacin, riboflavin, and pantothenic acid all play a critical role in thermogenesis due to their involvement in energy metabolism; however, there is no evidence at this time to support increased intake in the cold of any of these nutrients above MRDA (AR 40-25, 1985) levels. Evidence from studies conducted primarily in laboratory animals has suggested a role for the micronutrients iron, copper, and zinc in nonshivering thermogenesis. There is no evidence at this time to indicate that short-term depletion of any of these micronutrients interferes with thermoregulation in humans; however, more research is needed.

The macronutrient sources of energy (carbohydrate, protein, and fat) also have thermogenic effects. Fat is absorbed slowly but has the lowest postprandial thermogenic effect. Carbohydrates are absorbed most rapidly, but their thermogenic effect is higher and may last for 2 to 3 hours. Protein digestion gives rise to amino acids, which are absorbed more slowly than carbohydrates, but have the highest thermogenic effect, lasting up to 5 to 6 hours after absorption. The use of a high protein snack prior to retiring to sleep has been recommended to aid in thermoregulation.

9. Does the timing of food ingestion influence cold tolerance?

Postprandially induced thermogenesis can be a significant source of heat production within the body. Consumption of a substantial meal high in protein may provide necessary heat during periods of low activity or during sleep (see LeBlanc, Chapter 12 in this volume and the answer to Question 8 above). The consumption of small meals or snacks at intervals throughout periods of moderate activity is useful for maintaining body heat and work performance.

10. What is the relationship between fluid intake and thermoregulation in the cold and at altitude?

With acute exposure to both cold and high altitudes, fluid losses may result in a hypohydrated state. Diuresis is a common consequence of acute exposure to both conditions. Additional water is lost to the dry air through respiration, especially with the hyperventilation of exercise. Body water loss is also increased through sweating, especially if the individual is wearing excess clothing and engages in physical activity. Finally, fluid intake is often limited under these circumstances because of the response to stress, lack of fluid availability, or desire to control urine formation. The resulting reduction in body water, including blood and plasma volume, will decrease the ability to sweat. Thermoregulation is also affected by a decrease in body water due to the decrease in body heat transfer to the periphery with the decrease in blood volume because it is the blood that carries the body heat to the periphery, where it is given up to the environment through evaporative heat loss. Body fluid losses of greater than 10 percent of total body water are life threatening.

Some of this lost water will be replaced with metabolic water which is produced in greatest amounts with the burning of carbohydrate, the fuel of choice at altitude, and a fuel of significance in the cold. In spite of this, water balance is difficult to attain at altitude or in the cold due to the excessive losses, and the difficulties in supply.

11. What is the effect of cold and altitude exposure (at rest) on basal energy requirements?

Exposure to either cold or high altitudes significantly increases the energy needs of the body. In both cases, basal energy needs[2] (BMR) are elevated by as

---

[2] Basal metabolic rate (BMR) refers to a parameter measured under strict circumstances of temperature, time at rest, and nutritional status. Consequently the determination of metabolic rate in cold environments does not meet the definition of BMR. The term "basal energy needs" is used here to indicate the energy requirements of individuals in the cold,

much as 15 percent after acclimatization. In the cold, this elevation in energy requirements is consequent to the need to maintain body temperature. The cause of the increase at altitude is not as clearly defined but may be associated with the increased respiratory rate and difficulty in sleeping.

During acute exposure to high altitudes, both the magnitude and time frame of changes in the BMR will vary with total energy intake and environmental conditions. Generally, the BMR increases by 20 to 40 percent over BMR during the first days at high altitudes, and then falls somewhat over the ensuing 3 to 10 days. There may be some loss of lean body mass during this time period, occurring simultaneously with inadequate energy intake, as BMR begins to decline toward the level that existed prior to altitude exposure. In experiments where energy intake has been matched to increased needs, basal needs remain elevated throughout the time spent at high altitudes. Individuals who are native to high-altitude environments show an elevated basal energy requirement in comparison to low-altitude natives of similar body size. The basal energy needs of soldiers can, therefore, be expected to be elevated in cold, high-altitude environments.

Nutritional Requirements

12. What are typical energy requirements for work in cold and in high-altitude environments?

Work in the cold or at high altitudes may result in very high energy requirements. When doubly labeled water techniques were used to determine energy expenditures, mean total energy requirements of 3,400 to 4,300 kcal/d (or 2.5 to 3 times BMR) were recorded in sedentary male military personnel in the cold or at high altitudes. Under training conditions, the energy requirements increased to as much as 5,000 kcal/d. The individual requirement will depend on body size, clothing, and activity level, but energy requirements of 54 to 62/kcal/kg/d are recommended for these environments. Individual requirements may reach as much as 4 to 7 times BMR for short periods of time, especially when activities are being performed in clothing that restricts movement. No available studies define the total energy requirements during military operations under conditions of both intense cold and high altitudes. It should be noted, however, that there is no evidence that the actual energy expenditure of the work done is increased under the conditions of altitude exposure, although the hobbling effect of working in protective gear in the cold may increase appreciably the energy expended in given activities.

---

unrelated to exercise or the thermic effects of food. Determination of basal energy needs at altitude met the criteria for measurement of BMR.

13. Does cold or altitude exposure alter the requirement for nutrients other than energy?

With the possible exception of vitamin E, there appears to be little scientific basis at this time to indicate that cold or altitude exposure changes the nutritional requirements for any vitamins or minerals. Questions have been raised about increased needs for vitamin C, iron, zinc, and copper in cold and in high-altitude environments. The MRDAs for operational rations (AR 40-25, 1985) supply generous amounts of nutrients over the requirements in normal conditions and should be adequate to meet any small increases in requirements due to cold or altitude.

14. What is the sodium requirement for hard physical work in a cold environment?

Sodium requirements in the cold have not been the subject of specific investigation. Although there has been monitoring of sodium status in individuals participating in metabolic research in cold environments, the focus of these studies was not to determine sodium requirements, and thus dietary intake of sodium was not controlled.

There is good reason to conduct research on sodium requirements in cold environments especially where hard physical work is required. Excessively high sodium intake can lead to increased diuresis, which is a major concern in cold environments. On the other hand, it is well known that significant sodium loss can occur during heavy physical activity. This loss of sodium through sweating occurs in cold-weather conditions when body heat is allowed to build up in heavy clothing. The loss will likely be reduced after acclimatization occurs. In the absence of more data, it is recommended that sodium intake be maintained as recommended in the MRDAs with no additional amounts given for hard physical activity. It is unlikely that electrolyte complications will occur, such as those associated with hard physical work in hot environments.

15. What is the relationship between fluid intake and food intake in the cold or at altitude?

Requirements for food are clearly distinct and separate from requirements for water, even though some foods may partially satisfy water requirements and generate metabolic water after they are consumed. The distinction between needs for water and food is most evident in hot, arid desert-like conditions, where water needs are greatly increased because much body water is lost by physiological mechanisms used to maintain normal body temperatures. This distinction is equally necessary for working in cold and in high-altitude environments.

Extremes of both cold and high-altitude environments have independent effects upon the nutritional and physiological requirements for food and water. As detailed in several chapters (for example, see Chapters 7, 10, and 11 in this volume), physiological responses to extreme cold induce metabolic heat production, which in turn increases the need for an adequate intake of dietary energy. Cold stress also leads to dehydration because of cold-induced diuresis, a phenomenon stimulated by several possible physiologic mechanisms (see review in Chapter 1 in this volume). Body water losses are also increased in the cold because of increased losses of respiratory water as well as losses induced by sweating. Cold conditions tend to reduce fluid intake because of logistical difficulties in supplying water and in preventing it from freezing. Water discipline is as important during cold stress as it is during heat stress.

The pair of problems created in meeting food and fluid needs is exaggerated when high-altitude stress is superimposed upon cold stress. Fluid needs become complicated by physiologic processes and hormonal effects that induce an antidiuretic effect in some individuals (see Anand and Chandrashekhar, Chapter 18 in this volume). This effect can contribute to AMS as well as to high-altitude pulmonary edema. More commonly, however, dehydration may become a potential military problem. Dehydration can result from several causes (see Cymerman, Chapter 16 in this volume), including reduced thirst, inadequate fluid intakes (from both water and foods), and increased sensible and insensible water losses associated with exercise. Again, water discipline is a military necessity.

Increased energy needs are also a separate but important issue at high altitudes. Weight loss is a common reality that must be met by increasing fuel intakes to meet additional energy needs (see Butterfield, Chapter 19 in this volume). Dehydration may also result in anorectic symptoms and lowered food intake. The provision of high calorie, energy dense snack-type foods was recommended by several participants in this workshop and by the CMNR in a previous report (IOM, 1995) as a potential means of providing extra food energy. Thus, the needs for supplying fluids and for supplying food must each be approached as equally important, and logistical support for cold and high-altitude work in the military must take into consideration the distinct differences in effort that are required for the adequate provision of each.

These issues can be summarized in two general questions:

1. Aside from increased energy demands, do cold or high-altitude environments elicit an increased demand or requirement for specific nutrients?

Cold and/or high-altitude environments can increase the needs for two important nutrients, water and carbohydrate (see answers to Questions 2, 5, 8, 10, and 15 in this chapter). Additional fat may sometimes be required to supply energy needs under certain circumstances (see reply to Question 4). While preliminary studies of increasing vitamin E intake to 400 mg/d show research promise in providing protective effects at high altitudes, considerable additional research is needed before questions regarding efficacy and effective doses are fully addressed and before implementing a supplement policy (see reply to Question 6). The needs for certain other single nutrients, i.e., vitamin C, iron, zinc, copper, and sodium, may also be increased (see comments on Questions 7, 13, and 14), but because currently available data are inadequate, additional research will be needed to identify and define any increased needs for these nutrients. There is no evidence at this point to indicate a need for any of the nutrients to be provided at levels beyond that included in the MRDAs. For further elaboration see Chapter 1.

2. Can performance be enhanced in cold or high-altitude environments by the provision of increased amounts of specific nutrients?

Very little research is available to support any need to administer single nutrient dietary supplements in cold or high-altitude environments. As noted in an earlier CMNR report on *Food Components to Enhance Performance* (IOM, 1994), a number of nutrients have been investigated for these purposes but rarely under environmental conditions of cold or high altitudes. Harris R. Lieberman and his colleagues at the U.S. Army Research Institute of Environmental Medicine (USARIEM) have investigated single dose tyrosine pretreatment (100 mg/kg) in humans subjected to a 4.5-h exposure to cold and hypoxia. In a single controlled study, this large supplement significantly decreased symptoms, adverse moods, and performance impairments (Banderet and Lieberman, 1989). This work has been further expanded in several studies by the Naval Research group (Ahlers et al., 1994; Shurtleff et al., 1994). In rats, tyrosine pretreatment (400 mg/kg) reversed the behavioral depression caused by a forced swim in cold water, although it had no influence on deep body cooling (Rauch and Lieberman, 1990). These preliminary findings are worthy of additional future studies.

RECOMMENDATIONS

On the basis of the papers presented by the invited speakers, discussion at the workshop, and subsequent committee deliberations, the Committee on Military Nutrition Research offers the following recommendations regarding nutrient requirements for work in cold and in high-altitude environments.

Water and Dehydration

• Because cold-induced dehydration can cause serious performance decrements, it must be anticipated. The **training of military personnel assigned to cold-weather operations must include water discipline, safe fluid sources because snow or ice are generally unsafe, and the protection of drinking fluids from freezing.**

• Water discipline is as important during military operations in intense cold and at high altitudes as it is during desert heat. **Training should include water discipline measures following guidelines in military doctrines and means for their enforcement.**

Energy and Specific Nutrients

• Because of increased energy demands of cold operations, **dietary energy sources must be adequate to meet actual or anticipated needs,** including the needs for adequate carbohydrate foods. A field feeding doctrine, as previously recommended (IOM, 1995), should be considered. Pre-exposure diets should insure that muscle glycogen stores become optimized. **Meal times should be standardized whenever possible in order to encourage increased food intake.**

• **Carbohydrate intake should be promoted** during military operations conducted in the cold or at high altitudes. The inclusion of a liquid or solid carbohydrate supplement in the rations of troops may be useful in maintaining macronutrient balance and performance over time. **Carbohydrate intake should be at least 400g/d** under these conditions. When energy expenditures are high and total caloric intake is increased, the CMNR recommends that carbohydrate intake be increased to maintain calories from carbohydrate in the range of at least 40 percent of total caloric intake. This will help provide a palatable diet that is not excessive in fat content.

The Ration, Cold Weather (RCW), MRE, and LRP I as currently prescribed for cold-weather operations all provide a minimum of 4,300 kcal and 582 g carbohydrate per day (see Table 1-4). The percentages of calories in these rations that are contributed by carbohydrate are 49 percent for the MRE, 60 percent for the RCW, and 50 percent for the LRP I. Thus these all meet the recommended criteria.

• **Restriction of fat calories to only 30 percent,** as recommended for the American civilian population, **is not appropriate for some military operational rations** where caloric density, ration bulk, and palatability are of concern. This is particularly the case for rations designed for use in cold and in high-altitude environments. The percentages of calories in currently available rations that are contributed by fat are 36 percent for the MRE, 32 percent for the RCW, and 35 percent for the LRP I. These levels appear appropriate, given the situational requirements.

• Sharing of food rations is encouraged as a means of meeting the higher than average caloric needs of some individuals in the field.

• In the absence of more data concerning sodium requirements during heavy exercise in conditions of arctic cold, **normal sodium intakes should be maintained.**

Education and Logistics

• Because **physiologic responses and adaptations differ importantly between moderately high altitudes (8,000–12,000 ft [2,438–3,658 m]) and extremely high altitudes** (greater than 18,000 ft [5,486 m]), **planning for military training or military missions at high altitudes should take these differences into account.**

• **Individuals who have not yet regained lean body mass lost in prior field operations should not be deployed to cold or high-altitude environments until lean body mass is regained.**

• **Military troops, leaders, and medical personnel being assigned to high-altitude training or missions should be fully instructed on the symptoms and signs of AMS,** subacute mountain sickness, high-altitude pulmonary edema **(HAPE),** and high-altitude cerebral edema **(HACE).** In addition, they should be trained in the use of appropriate countermeasures and therapy.

Because about 25 percent of people seem to be "immune" to AMS, **military personnel who have successfully completed a tour at altitude should be the ones selected for assignment to altitude missions of unique military importance.** Conversely, those who have developed AMS during training at high altitudes should be excluded in advance from participating in such unique military missions whenever possible.

• **Information about possible changes in physical performance, alertness, and emotional stability associated with hypoxia should be provided** to all levels of command so that soldiers and their leaders will not be surprised when they occur. Breakdown in troop cohesion should be anticipated.

• Because weight loss is common during military operations at high altitudes, command and logistical practices should attempt to ensure, whenever possible, that **the availability of palatable foods and fluids, as well as the social setting at mealtimes, are optimized to insure adequate dietary intakes** (see IOM, 1995).

• Logistical measures for cold-weather operations must put primary emphasis on the delivery and maintenance of sufficient food stores and unfrozen dietary fluids.

• Military rations are the fuel for the soldier and emphasis should be placed on adequate availability and consumption of operational rations to maintain performance in these harsh environments.

AREAS FOR FUTURE RESEARCH

The Committee on Military Nutrition Research suggests a number of areas for future research within the military related to nutrition for soldiers working in cold and in high-altitude environments. The CMNR believes that the military services, through their pool of volunteer personnel, offer an excellent and often unique opportunity to generate research data and statistics on the nutrition, health, and well-being of service personnel. It is important that future studies include men and women representative of the full range of ages in the active duty military. These findings can be directly applied to improve both the health of military personnel and that of the general U.S. population.

Water and Dehydration

Further research is needed:

• to define the best strategies (including pharmacological ones) to avoid cold-induced dehydration.
• to define the water needs of the body during the early phases of exposure to high altitudes, along with its relationship to the diuresis experienced by many subjects, and importantly, to the development of acute mountain illnesses.
• to define the potential "value" of dehydration in association with long-term stays at moderate altitudes and to define the limits whereby such dehydration might be preventable, beneficial, or detrimental.

Energy

Further research is needed:

• to assess the applicability to the military, both men and women, of the finding that it may be possible to maintain body weight, nitrogen balance, and muscle protein mass at optimal values during high-altitude missions.
• to define energy requirements during military operations in which simultaneous exposures to intense cold and high altitudes occur, by validation of the "free-living" estimation of energy requirement based on Hoyt and Honig's proposed use of body weight, foot strike, and terrain (see Chapter 20 in this volume).
• to understand the metabolic aspects of shivering.

Specific Nutrients

Further research is needed:

• to define more precisely the carbohydrate intake required to maintain body glycogen stores and to replenish stores depleted by exercise in the cold and at high altitudes.

• to establish whether a specific proportion of calories from fat, carbohydrate, or protein has a clear-cut advantage in maintaining thermoregulation in cold environments.

• to determine the optimum intake of micronutrients for improving performance in the cold. Such studies must control for nutrient status prior to and at the time of testing, the training level of subjects, and intensity and duration of any exercise to be tested.

• to determine sodium requirements during heavy exercise in intensely cold conditions and the possible advantages of restricting sodium during the first few days at altitude.

• to determine the possible beneficial effects of anorexia at altitude.

• to determine whether supplemental doses of vitamin E have any protective effects on humans exposed to oxidative stress.

• to determine if supplements of vitamin C, iron, zinc, copper, and/or other nutrients could improve performance during the stresses of extreme cold and high altitudes.

Performance and Medical Conditions

Further research is needed:

• to explore the merits of some potentially useful pharmacological compounds such as theophylline, caffeine, and ephedrine, as well as the potential value of prestress tyrosine administration.

• to evaluate possible pharmacological, physiological, and nutritional methods, either in the field or in altitude chambers, to predict, prevent, and/or treat AMS.

• to consider the pathophysiological problems of salt and water balance and the intercompartmental shifts in body fluids at altitude. Physiological mechanisms requiring additional study include cardiovascular, renal, endocrine, metabolic, and biochemical responses.

• to resolve conflicting data on possible effects of cold exposure on muscle strength and endurance.

• to examine the relationship between the aging process and acclimatization. Research in this area would not only be beneficial to the military but the general American population.

• to improve the understanding of mood and performance changes over time in subjects exposed to high altitudes and hypoxia, using animal models for the purpose of identifying the neurochemical cause(s) of those changes.

• to develop follow-up drug and nutrient intervention strategies for ameliorating chemical changes, and thus, ideally mood and performance decrements at high altitudes.

• to develop and evaluate diet-focused pharmacologic countermeasures (e.g., tyrosine and caffeine), with the ultimate goal of applying such countermeasures in field situations to stem the decline in cognitive function that accompanies the exposure to adverse environmental conditions.

• to define the effects of acclimatization to high altitudes in terms of altered performance measures and to optimize nutrition for more rapid acclimatization.

• to address the impact of preexisting malnutrition on the performance of soldiers at environmental extremes of cold and altitude, possibly through the use of key nutrient deficiency screening procedures to be administered to individuals prior to their participation in unique military missions or training in the cold and at high altitudes.

Military Ration Development and Guidance

Further research is needed:

• to insure that consumption of rations specially developed by the Army for use in cold-weather conditions provides intakes of energy, protein, and micronutrients that fully meet the increased requirements of troops operating in the field.

• to optimize packaging, delivery, and serving of these rations to insure that adequate amounts are consumed.

SUMMARY

In summary, the CMNR wants to emphasize the critical importance of water discipline, availability of safe fluids for drinking, and a clear understanding on the part of all troops involved in operations or training in cold and in high-altitude environments. High energy, palatable rations supplying at least 400 g carbohydrate per day must be provided to insure that energy intake matches energy expenditure. Restriction of fat calories to only 30 percent is not appropriate in these operational rations. All military personnel who participate in cold and in high-altitude operations or training must be well informed about the symptoms and signs of AMS, HAPE, HACE, and possible changes in physical and cognitive performance, and trained in appropriate countermeasures. The logistics of troop supply and the composition of cold and high-altitude military units should be carefully screened regarding their previous experiences in these environments and their current nutritional and overall health status. Individuals who have not yet regained lean body mass lost in prior field operations should not be deployed to cold or high-altitude environments until lean body mass is regained.

An impressive body of evidence has already been generated to define the nutritional needs of troops required to engage in military operations under environmental conditions of extreme cold and/or high altitudes. The chapters in this report have addressed a number of specific nutritional areas and unanswered questions that need additional research study. The preceding series of research recommendations stem from these apparent gaps in knowledge. These informational gaps or uncertainties must be resolved in order to help define nutritional needs and military logistic strategies most appropriate for operations under these environmental extremes.

The primary nutritional considerations for soldiers operating in the cold or at high altitudes are:

• Fluid intake must be encouraged to prevent dehydration. Water discipline as practiced in hot, dry environments should be applied to operations in the cold and at high altitudes.

• Individuals who have not yet regained lean body mass lost in prior field operations should not be deployed to cold or high-altitude environments until lean body mass is regained.

• Energy intake of soldiers is usually inadequate when operating in the cold or at high altitudes. The deficit in intake frequently observed at moderate climates may be increased due to the greater energy needs when operating in these environments. Encouragement of food intake, use of supplemental rations, and alteration of energy composition through modest increases in fat content (to no more than 40 percent of total caloric intake) may aid but not fully overcome the deficit in intake usually observed in these environments.

• Increased carbohydrate intake (to at least 400 g/d) when functioning at higher altitudes is recommended to help maintain soldier performance.

• There appears to be little scientific evidence to indicate that cold or altitude exposure should change the nutritional allowances for any vitamins or minerals, with the possible exception of increased needs for vitamin E at high altitudes beyond that recommended for military rations. Further studies may be required to evaluate the suggestion that the needs for iron, zinc, copper, and vitamin C are influenced by cold temperatures. Carefully controlled studies are needed to evaluate whether or not supplemental doses of vitamin E have any protective function at high altitudes.

• Several areas for additional research have been identified that may offer future benefits in improving performance under the environmental extremes of cold or high altitudes. Among those most critical to military operations are (1) the need to define further the water requirements in cold and in high-altitude environments, and how best to meet them; (2) the need to apply to military personnel the recent findings concerning maintenance of body weight and composition at altitude by encouraging the intake of a minimum level of dietary carbohydrate and total calories; (3) the need to determine the optimal ratio of energy sources, micronutrients, and sodium in the cold; (4) the need to develop better methods to predict, prevent, and treat altitude-related illnesses; and finally (5) the need to obtain a better understanding of the causes, ramifications, and treatments of altitude-related changes in mood and performance.

The Committee on Military Nutrition Research is pleased to participate with the Military Nutrition Division, U.S. Army Research Institute of Environmental Medicine and U.S. Army Medical Research and Materiel Command in programs related to the nutrition and health of American military personnel. The CMNR hopes that this information will be useful and helpful to the Department of Defense in developing programs that continue to improve the lifetime health and well-being of service personnel.

REFERENCES

Ahlers, S.T., J.R. Thomas, J. Schrot, and D. Shurtleff. 1994. Tyrosine and glucose modulation of cognitive deficits resulting from cold stress. Pp. 301–320 in Food Components to Enhance Performance, An Evaluation of Potential Performance-Enhancing Food Components for Operational Rations, B.M. Marriott, ed. A report of the Committee on Military Nutrition Research, Food and Nutrition Board, Institute of Medicine. Washington, D.C.: National Academy Press.

AR (Army Regulation) 40-25. 1985. *See* U.S. Departments of the Army, the Navy, and the Air Force.

Askew, E.W. 1995. Environmental and physical stress and nutrient requirements. Am. J. Clin. Nutr. 61(suppl.):631S–637S.

Baker-Fulco, C.J. 1995. An overview of dietary intakes during military exercises. Pp. 121–149 in Not Eating Enough, Overcoming Underconsumption of Military Operational Rations, B.M. Marriott, ed. A report of the Committee on Military Nutrition Research, Food and Nutrition Board, Institute of Medicine. Washington, D.C.: National Academy Press.

Banderet, L.E., and H.R. Lieberman. 1989. Treatment with tyrosine, a neurotransmitter precursor, reduces environmental stress in humans. Brain Res. Bull. 22:759–762.

Bendich, A., and Machlin, L.J. 1988. Safety of oral intake of vitamin E. Am. J. Clin. Nutr. 48:612–619.

Brooks, G.A., G.E. Butterfield, R.R. Wolfe, B.M. Groves, R.S. Mazzeo, J.R. Sutton, E.E. Wolfel, and J.T. Reeves. 1991. Increased dependence on blood glucose after acclimatization to 4,300 m. J. Appl. Physiol. 70:919–927.

CDC (Centers for Disease Control and Prevention). 1994. Daily dietary fat and total food energy intakes—Third National Health and Nutrition Examination Survey. Phase 1, 1989–91. Morbid. Mortal. Weekly Rep. 43(7):116–125.

Consolazio F.C., L.O. Matoush, H.L. Johnson, H.J. Krzywicki, T.A. Daws, and G.J. Isaac. 1969. Effects of high-carbohydrate diets on performance and clinical symptomatology after rapid ascent to high altitude. Fed. Proc. 28:937–943.

Edwards, J.S.A., and D.E. Roberts. 1991. The influence of a calorie supplement on the composition of the Meal, Ready-to-Eat in a cold environment. Milit. Med. 156:466–471.

Edwards, J.S.A., D.E. Roberts, and S.H. Mutter. 1992. Rations for use in a cold environment. J. Wilderness Med. 3:27–47.

IOM (Institute of Medicine). 1994. Food Components to Enhance Performance, An Evaluation of Potential Performance-Enhancing Food Components for Operational Rations. A report of the Committee on Military Nutrition Research, Food and Nutrition Board. Washington, D.C.: National Academy Press.

IOM. 1995. Not Eating Enough, Overcoming Underconsumption of Military Operational Rations. A report of the Committee on Military Nutrition Research, Food and Nutrition Board. Washington, D.C.: National Academy Press.

King, N., M.R. Sutherland, S.H. Mutter, E.W. Askew, and D.E. Roberts. 1993. Cold weather field evaluation of the 18-Man Arctic Tray Pack Ration Module, the Meal, Ready-to-Eat, and the Long Life Ration Packet. Milt. Med. 158:458–465.

Kleiber, M. 1961. The Fire of Life. New York: John Wiley and Sons.

LeBlanc, J. 1957. Effect of environmental temperature on energy expenditure and calorie requirements. J. Appl. Physiol. 10:281–283.

NRC (National Research Council). 1989. Recommended Dietary Allowances, 10th ed. A report of the Subcommittee on the Tenth Edition of the RDAs, Food and Nutrition Board. Washington, D.C.: National Academy Press.

Panin, L.E., N.M. Mayaskaya, A.A. Borodin et al. 1992. Comparison of biochemical reactions to trek and chamber simulations. Pp. 139–186 in Observations on the Soviet/Canadian Transpolar Ski Trek. Basel, Switzerland: Karger.

Rauch, T.M., and H.R. Lieberman. 1990. Pre-treatment with tyrosine reverses hypothermia induced behavioral depression. Brain Res. Bull. 24:147–150.

Roberts, A.C., G.E. Butterfield, J.T. Reeves, E.E. Wolfel, and G.A. Brooks. In Press a. Acclimatization to 4,300 m altitude decreases reliance on fat as a substrate. J. Appl. Physiol.

Roberts, A.C., J.T. Reeves, G.E. Butterfield, R.S. Mazzeo, J.R. Sutton, E.E. Wolfel, and G.A. Brooks. In Press b. Altitude and B-Blockade augment glucose utilization during exercise. J. Appl. Physiol.

Shurtleff, D., J.R. Thomas, J. Schrot, K. Kowalski, and R. Harford. 1994. Tyrosine reverses a cold-induced memory deficiency in humans. Pharmacol. Biochem. Behav. 47:935–941.

Simon-Schnass, I. 1992. Nutrition at high altitude. J. Nutr. 122:778–781.

Swain, H.L., F.M. Toth, F.C. Consolazio, W.H. Fitzpatrick, D.I. Allen, and C.J. Koehn. 1949. Food consumption of soldiers in a subarctic climate. J. Nutr. 38:63–72.

USDA (U.S. Department of Agriculture). 1995. Report of the Dietary Guidelines Advisory Committee on the Dietary Guidelines for Americans, 1995. Washington, D.C.: Government Printing Office.

U.S. Departments of the Army, the Navy, and the Air Force. 1985. Army Regulation 40-25/Naval Command Medical Instruction 10110.1/Air Force Regulation 160-95. "Nutrition Allowances, Standards, and Education." May 15. Washington, D.C.

Appendix G

Conclusions and Recommendations from the Brief Report Pennington Biomedical Research Center September 1996 Site Visit

Submitted September 1996

Conclusions and Recommendations

GENERAL COMMENTS

The committee continues to be impressed with the excellence of the facility at the PBRC for laboratory and clinical research. Continued progress has been made in the staffing of this large facility. The laboratories are extremely well-equipped for research in the areas of the Army's interests. The equipment for supporting this research program has largely been provided by a USDA grant. Financial support for the research activities has progressed significantly, with funds provided by the U.S. Army, USDA, NIH, and various other sources. George A. Bray, M.D., director of the PBRC, and Donna H. Ryan, M.D., principal investigator for the military nutrition grant, have effectively recruited a qualified staff to conduct the research outlined in the Army grant. The scientific and administrative direction appear to be solid. It is the committee's judgment that as the PBRC receives new directives from its military sponsor, the center now has the staff and expertise to develop appropriate programs utilizing its individual laboratory units as interactive modules. The PBRC has noted that the center's military nutrition research goals for 1997–2002 are: to increase publications, patents, and technology transfer; to increase collaboration with Army scientists; to increase the integration of specific tasks and laboratories; to conduct a military nutrition symposium every other year; and to invite a "military nutrition visiting professor" six times yearly for consultation and peer review.

SPECIFIC PROJECT REVIEWS[1]

Overview of Project Tasks

As described in the introduction, the PBRC is requesting funding for an additional 5 years to conduct research concerning issues of nutrition relevant to the military. The research as outlined in the preproposal consists of the following:

- measuring energy and water needs of troops in the field,
- providing laboratory support for field studies,
- providing nutrition assessment support in field studies,
- enhancing the nutrition of military menus, and
- developing nutritional strategies for improved military performance under stressful conditions.

A total of nine specific projects were developed by the PBRC to meet the U.S. Army objectives. These specific tasks that the CMNR were asked to review include:

- Clinical Laboratory for Human and Food Samples (Task 1),
- Stable Isotope Laboratory (Task 2),
- Stress, Nutrition, and Mental Performance (Task 3),
- Stress, Sleep Deprivation, and Performance (Task 4),
- Stress, Nutrition, and Work Performance (Task 5),
- Menu Modification/Enhancing Military Diet Project (Task 6),
- Nutrient Database Integration Laboratory (Task 7),
- Stress, Nutrition, and Immune Function Laboratory (Task 8), and
- Metabolic Unit Projects.

Task 1: Clinical Laboratory for Human and Food Samples

Project Summary

This project is headed by Richard T. Tully, Ph.D., with major assistance from Jennifer C. Rood, Ph.D. The primary function of this laboratory under the U.S. Army grant is to provide nutrition laboratory research support to the military nutrition research program at USARIEM. This support includes performing biochemical assessment of nutritional status and performing analyses of nutrient and biochemical substances in foods used in military rations

---

[1] Please note that the task numbers correspond to the task numbers assigned in the preproposal (see Appendix II).

and clinical studies. This laboratory is the central laboratory responsible for analyzing blood, urine, stool, tissue, and food samples. In the future, the laboratory proposes in-field computerized data processing of samples to speed processing time, as well as establishing a database that would be accessible to many Army facilities.

General Comments

This review of the laboratory's operation reveals that Dr. Tully and his staff are well qualified and knowledgeable about the wide range of analytical methods required to support the research program. The procedures used for sample transportation, receipt, storage, preparation, and analysis are clearly defined. Sample analyses are accomplished in a timely manner to meet USARIEM's program needs. The laboratory has a sound quality assurance program and uses standard reference materials to check the adequacy of procedure performance. It is noted that the laboratory follows Good Laboratory Practices regulations and is accredited by the College of American Pathologists. It also is noted that additional method development is underway for tests needed for future research. For the size of its staff, the number of procedures currently being performed by the laboratory is very impressive.

The progress that has been made in rendering this laboratory fully operational is excellent. The laboratory houses state-of-the-art equipment and a well-trained staff. It is evident by the level of clinical laboratory support provided to USARIEM in conducting military nutrition research that this laboratory is vital to the DoD nutrition research program.

Specific Comments, Concerns, and Questions

The staff of the Clinical Research Laboratory has been consulting with the U.S. Department of Agriculture Food Composition Laboratory to obtain expertise in the accomplishment of food analysis. The committee agrees that this relationship is important and that such consultation should continue.

Recommendations

The committee suggests that the laboratory should facilitate additional contacts, such as with the FDA's Regional Laboratory in Atlanta, for nutrient analysis. In the area of clinical methods, it may be useful to establish a relationship with the laboratories at the Centers for Disease Control and Prevention in Atlanta. Participation in interlaboratory collaborative studies to verify new methods under the guidelines of the Association of Official Analytical Chemists is also recommended. These laboratories will provide guidance in the development and implementation of new laboratory tests that will best support the current clinical laboratory projects as well as in the development of the methodology required and proposed for food composition and analysis. As the Menu Modification/Enhancing Military Diets Project develops and broadens in scope, maintaining expertise in methodologic issues will be key.

The committee recommends that the additional expenditure of resources be permitted for the development and implementation of methods necessary for the assessment of immune function (in support of Task 8). The development of these methods will be coordinated by the immunologist who is directing the project on Stress and Immune Function (Task 8).

The committee recommends that efforts associated with expanding the capability of chemical analysis of food composition be restricted to obtaining data that are not available from other reliable sources and which directly support metabolic unit studies.

Finally, the committee recommends continued financial support of the Clinical Research Laboratory, as this laboratory provides services to the Stable Isotope Laboratory, Menu Modification/Enhancing Military Diets Project, and the Nutrient Database Integration Laboratory (see Tasks 1, 2, 6, and 7). Financial support should be maintained at a level consistent with USARIEM needs.

Task 2: Stable Isotope Laboratory

Project Summary

This project is directed by James P. DeLany, Ph.D., and involves the use of the doubly labeled water technique to determine energy expenditure in the field and total body water measurements to monitor changes in body composition. The work of this laboratory represents one of the major service functions of the PBRC for the Army. In the past funding period, the laboratory has been involved in 17 completed studies in collaboration with USARIEM, accomplishing 169 doubly labeled water, 222 water turnover, and 616 total body water determinations. At present, the laboratory is involved in analyses of samples from four additional studies conducted in conjunction with USARIEM.

General Comments

Although no specific new work is proposed in the preproposal presented to the CMNR, it is assumed that this laboratory will continue to be available to the Army on an "as needed" basis to complete similar kinds of measurements in studies yet to be specified.

Dr. DeLany has been funded by the Defense Women's Health Research Program to evaluate total daily energy requirements and activity patterns in servicewomen performing a wide range of tasks.

Dr. DeLany indicated that new equipment had been ordered for the laboratory (and is due for delivery) to allow for an increased volume and variety of analyses to be conducted. This equipment will expand the capability of the laboratory to assist in the conduct of studies on various metabolic pathways, such as protein turnover, muscle protein synthesis, and metabolic fuel use during exercise, which could be done in conjunction with other studies proposed to meet the needs of the military (see Tasks 5 and 8).

Specific Comments and Concerns

The lack of integration between this laboratory and others that was suggested by the preproposal is disturbing to the CMNR. Given the directions proposed by other investigators in that preproposal, there are several opportunities for collaboration. These would include investigations such as the ones proposed under Tasks 5 and 8, to determine protein requirements and turnover as well as fuel use and the optimal type of fuel under conditions of intense physical stress that impact on immune function.

Recommendations

The committee recommends that the Stable Isotope Laboratory continue in its service function to assist the Army in its on-going research program. In addition, Dr. DeLany and coworkers should continue to assist the Army with developing experimental designs that ensure the optimal execution of studies using doubly labeled water as well as other stable isotopes. The committee believes that to date this facility has been underutilized, and ample opportunity exists for greater collaboration within the PBRC. The funding of this laboratory should be consistent with the level required to support the Army's nutrition research program.

Task 3: Stress, Nutrition, and Mental Performance

Project Summary

The basic project, headed by Ruth B. S. Harris, Ph.D., involves studies of the impact of stress on neurochemical and behavioral indices of performance using a rodent model. This line of investigation has developed from an interest in ascertaining how stress modifies brain chemistry and function, with the goal of designing appropriate nutritional and pharmacologic strategies to ameliorate the adverse effects of stress. A number of behavioral, nutritional, sensory, and neurochemical findings have been documented, some of which are being prepared for publication and many of which suggest productive future avenues to pursue.

Rodent models have been developed to evaluate the impact of nutritional interventions for their potential to moderate or prevent stress-induced neurochemical changes and their subsequent behavioral deficits. Many models have been evaluated, including a model of acute stress; a model of chronic stress induced by sleep deprivation or by restraint; chronic mild stress induced by exposure to a random mild stressor for several weeks; and an alternate model to study stress and retention utilizing a fixed-ratio training schedule in operant chambers. The stress models currently in use by the Nutritional Neuroscience Laboratory include a chronic stress and an acute stress model. The chronic stress model utilizes 4 days of Rapid Eye Movement sleep deprivation (REMd) to induce a state of stress. The acute stress model measures the effect of either 3 hours of restraint in a small cylinder or immobilization restraint for 30 minutes to 3 hours. This apparatus is a cylindrical enclosure attached to one side of an open field. A rat is placed inside the chamber, and the time to leave the chamber, number of reentries, total time in the chamber, and locomotor activity in the open field are recorded.

The studies proposed for the renewal project period continue several of the earlier lines of investigation into the mechanisms and effects of stress, in addition to a new project entitled "Genetic Markers for Stress Susceptibility" to investigate the interaction of stress and genetic background in the rodent model. A variety of strategies will be used to identify potential candidate genes.

General Comments

This laboratory has had changes in leadership since it was first established 6 years ago. Under the current leadership of Ruth B. S. Harris, Ph.D., significant progress has been made toward the aims proposed in the last project submission (see Appendix III).

While some of the laboratory's approaches will no doubt yield interesting outcomes, the committee feels that some focus is needed owing to the complexity of stress as a physiologic phenomenon and to the various techniques that have been used to evaluate the stress response experimentally.

Specific Comments, Concerns, and Questions

Specifically, the committee believes that a re-evaluation is needed of the models of stress being examined, so as to focus on one or two models that have the greatest potential relevance to the military mission. Once identified, these models should be examined behaviorally, neurochemically, pharmacologically, and nutritionally to identify vulnerable brain functions and potential countermeasures. Unless such an approach is taken, there is the possibility that this important area of investigation will remain unfocused, and thus unlikely to lead to the important insights regarding stress and mental function that are necessary to improve human performance under stressful military conditions.

Recommendations

The committee recommends that the investigators seek expert help in stress, pharmacology, and formulation of research diets to assist in the identification of appropriate pharmacologic and nutritional models and interventions. This may be accomplished in conjunction with the PBRC's 1997–2002 research goals as presented at the site visit, one of which is to bring in visiting professors; it may also be accomplished by holding a 1-day meeting specifically dedicated to examining animal models of stress, that have been used successfully in measuring stress. Speakers would evaluate models of stress with which they are familiar in the context of the stresses experienced in the military.

The committee strongly believes that the PBRC investigators must seek a model which more appropriately fits the human experience of stress; with the use of this model, important insights may be gained regarding the manner by which stress compromises brain function, an issue of particular importance to the military mission. Such insights may ultimately lead to effective nutritional and pharmacological measures to combat the negative effects of stress in a military context. In addition, the committee believes that investigations attempting to identify the genes responsible for controlling the response to stress are premature as experienced investigators and facilities are lacking at this time.

Task 4: Stress, Sleep Deprivation, and Performance

Project Summary

This clinical project, as presented by George A. Bray, M.D.; Richard A. Magill, Ph.D.; and William F. Waters, Ph.D., involves studies in sleep deprived human subjects to ascertain whether chemical and nutritional interventions can minimize the cognitive deficits associated with sleep loss. The investigators have pursued these studies for several years, examining such agents as tyrosine, amphetamine, caffeine, and phentermine. The preliminary presentation of results during the site visit indicates that amphetamine clearly improved several of the cognitive deficits produced by sleep deprivation. Smaller effects were noted for phentermine and caffeine, while unremarkable effects were observed for tyrosine. As presented, the results are consistent with earlier findings for each agent and suggest that weak pharmacologic agents are not particularly potent in improving performance deficits associated with sleep loss.

A proposal has been made to continue this line of investigation and to examine the effect on performance of administering tyrosine alone or in combination with caffeine during a longer period of sleep deprivation. Another proposed study would compare the effects of tryptophan alone with that of tryptophan in combination with melatonin to evaluate whether these agents can improve sleep efficacy during short naps provided intermittently during the sleep deprivation period.

General Comments

At the time of this review, while a large number of studies were reported to have been completed, the data had not yet been thoroughly analyzed statistically.

Specific Comments, Concerns, and Questions

Overall, it would appear that this project has succeeded in fulfilling its mission: it has shown that caffeine may be useful as a nonprescription agent for enhancing performance during sleep deprivation, but that tyrosine is not.

Based on the data collected and analyzed to date, it appears that additional studies are unlikely to lead to new and potent intervention strategies using these agents. Hence, the need to continue such studies is not evident. The committee is aware of other, well-established neuroscience sleep laboratories within the military system that currently are working on similar projects.

Recommendations

The CMNR feels that it would <u>not</u> be in the Army's best interest to continue to provide support for the conduct of the sleep-deprivation studies within the Sleep Laboratory.

Task 6: Menu Modification/Enhancing Military Diets Project and Task 7: Nutrient Database Integration Laboratory

Project Summary

In its preproposal, the PBRC has divided the original Menu Modification Project into two projects. The newly named project, Enhancing Military Diets

Project, was initiated during September–October 1995 and will continue the recipe development activities using testing procedures similar to those developed for the previous project under the direction of Catherine Champagne, Ph.D. Chef Kelly Patrick has developed new recipes and has begun bench-top testing. The PBRC currently is assembling an acceptability panel that will consist of 50 to 100 panelists who fit the profile of U.S. military personnel to evaluate the recipes. Acceptability and consumption studies will follow at the Army Quartermaster Cooks School at Fort Lee, Virginia.

Past activities in the Menu Modification Project focused on the development of recipes to achieve the stated reduction in fat and cholesterol necessary to achieve the desired goals of no more than 30 percent of total calories from fat, and approximately 300 mg/d of cholesterol, for meals served in the Army garrison dining halls (A Rations). Forty-seven recipes have been tested for acceptability by panels at the PBRC and at Louisiana Tech. Similar methods of acceptability testing done at Fort Polk gave results comparable to those at Louisiana Tech, supporting the use of such nonmilitary panels to predict acceptability in an actual Army feeding situation. The lack of such comparable data was a concern expressed at the last CMNR site visit (see Appendix IV).

A 2-week study also was conducted at Fort Polk in which the new recipes were incorporated into dining hall menus during the second week. Data collected on food consumption in the dining hall plus food records for food consumed off base showed a significant reduction in fat intake (from 34.5 percent to 31.8 percent) with the modified menu compared to the regular menu for food eaten in the dining hall. It was noted, however, that approximately 50 percent of the food intake of personnel in Army facilities is from food consumed off base (outside of military dining facilities). The total fat consumed from these meals averaged 35.4 percent during each period of the study.

Based on interviews with Army personnel, PBRC investigators have proposed a list of modified recipes for testing, with an emphasis on ethnic foods and new breakfast items.

The new task proposed for the Nutrient Database Integration Laboratory involves the development and expansion of activities to assist the Army in estimation of the nutrient content of recipes and menus, as well as in the evaluation of dietary intake records from field studies conducted by USARIEM. Since 1989, the PBRC has participated in a support role in a number of studies. The Nutrient Data Systems Section at USARIEM has been involved in active data collection since 1993. In assessing military diets, a modified visual estimation method as well as food records have been utilized. In January 1995, the PBRC was approached by the Army sponsor to facilitate a more efficient form of collecting and disseminating dietary intake data from garrison and field studies. One such collaborative study which has been undertaken is the Savannah study conducted in July and August 1996. The leader of the data collection team for this project was Dr. Champagne, and the co-leader responsible for data entry was Ray Allen, Ph.D. A database system called MiDAS (Military Data Acquisition System) has been developed for use in the assessment of food intake in military settings. The PBRC staff will integrate all Armed Forces recipes, special formulations (Meals, Ready-to-Eat), and other food formulations into one centralized database system as part of this task.

General Comments for Tasks 6 and 7

In the letter report dated May 12, 1992, the CMNR noted several shortcomings in the Menu Modification Project. These included: (1) a lack of sensitivity to the needs of the military garrison feeding program, (2) inadequate evaluation procedures of modified menus, and (3) lack of interaction between the menu developers and the military menu system (see Appendix IV). The CMNR is pleased to note that PBRC investigators have overcome many of these shortcomings and have established working relationships with Army dietitians at USARIEM and with Army facilities such as Fort Polk and Fort Lee. Future activities with USARIEM include a visit of the PBRC team to the Army Quartermasters Cooks School at Fort Lee, Virginia to observe current training of Army cooks and a meeting with personnel responsible for determining the Army Master menu, as well as meeting with personnel responsible for food purchasing.

The proposed new leader of this project, Alana Cline, Ph.D., has extensive knowledge of military feeding systems and will facilitate further strengthening of the interactions of the PBRC with USARIEM. The past and proposed activities of this project are viewed as highly valuable by the Army and will make possible the accomplishment of tasks they currently are unable to do.

The Nutrient Database Integration Laboratory project will take advantage of the excellent PBRC computer facilities and expertise in dietary intake methodology to provide USARIEM with much-needed assistance in obtaining dietary data faster and more efficiently. Nutrient databases that have been incorporated into the PBRC database laboratory include the Bogalusa Heart Study and USDA Handbook 8 databases, as well as the Army's CAN (Computerized Analysis of Nutrients) database system. The PBRC nutrient database has been validated against the University of Minnesota Nutrition Coding Center database, and also has been utilized in two large, NIH-sponsored multicenter clinical trials.

Specific Comments, Concerns, and Questions for Tasks 6 and 7

Since it was demonstrated that approximately 50 percent of the food intake of personnel in Army facilities represents food consumed outside of military dining halls, it is questionable whether the development of low fat menus alone will achieve the goals of reducing total fat intake. However, any measurable reduction should be considered constructive, and those few individuals selecting all their meals in the military dining halls will benefit substantially.

There is additional concern regarding the micronutrient content of the modified menus. In particular, it is felt that additional attention must be focused on the levels of iron, calcium, zinc, folate, and vitamin B_6 (that is, micronutrients likely to be limiting when the use of ingredients from animal sources is curtailed in favor of lowering fat) provided by these dishes, in addition to the concern about their fat content.

Recommendations for Tasks 6 and 7

The CMNR recommends that estimation of plate waste be included in future field acceptability studies, such as the upcoming study at Fort Bliss, to provide for a more quantitative and qualitative assessment of dietary intakes.

In addition to menu modification, the committee strongly recommends to the PBRC and to the Army the use of nutritional education approaches such as those in the Army's Performance Power nutrition education program in order to achieve dietary intakes that meet military dietary goals.

The CMNR believes the Menu Modification/Enhancing Military Diets Project is relevant to the Army mission and provides valuable support to USARIEM. Since there are a number of nutrient databases in existence, it will be important to integrate these to avoid unnecessary duplication and to assure the integrity of this database. The proposed new task to develop the Nutrient Database Integration Laboratory is the next logical step in the development of a unified nutrition program that may facilitate the evaluation and comparison of dietary intake data with comparable data from the civilian sector at a later date.

Task 5: Stress, Nutrition, and Work Performance and
Task 8: Stress, Nutrition, and Immune Function Laboratory

Project Summary

As described by Jeffery J. Zachwieja, Ph.D., Task 5, entitled "Stress, Nutrition, and Work Performance," proposes to use outpatient volunteers to develop repeatable and reliable models to assess effects of carbohydrate delivery, amino acids, and caffeine on work performance and tolerance.

In addition, Dr. Zachwieja proposes to conduct studies using a rat model of stress. These rat studies, as described, will be closely integrated with Task 3 (Stress, Nutrition, and Mental Performance) of Ruth B. S. Harris, Ph.D., of the Nutritional Neuroscience Laboratory and with Task 8 of David W. Horohov, Ph.D., of the Stress, Nutrition, and Immune Function Laboratory. Descriptions of Dr. Horohov's task indicate that many, if not all, of his initial studies will be done in a rat model of stress in an attempt to develop a reproducible and predictable rat model for characterizing the mechanics of stress and immune dysfunction.

General Comments for Tasks 5 and 8

The committee believes that the integration of Tasks 5 and 8 is highly desirable but suggests that the objectives of both tasks would best be accomplished in human subjects. The superb PBRC Metabolic Unit would easily allow these performance studies to be conducted so that studies of balance, body composition, protein turnover, energy metabolism (these last three using stable isotopes), and immune function could all be combined and data obtained under closely controlled conditions. The independent variables would be physical activity and nutritional alterations (including modest-to-severe protein/energy deficiency as experienced in Ranger training). The integration of Tasks 5 and 8 will support a key directive from the Military Nutrition Division at USARIEM to test and evaluate nutrients and pharmacologic agents that may enhance performance. Such studies could build upon previous data obtained in Ranger trainees, as highlighted in previous CMNR publications (IOM, 1992, 1993). These studies documented the effects of demanding physical activity combined with limited food intake and limited sleep, which resulted in a 12 to 15 percent average weight loss over a period of about 9 weeks that was coupled with episodic increases in accidents and infections (IOM, 1993). This situation of low body fat, undernutrition, altered endocrine patterns, and perturbations in immune function suggested the need to develop important and practical nutritional countermeasures. Two important testable issues are whether improving the protein-to-energy ratio, under conditions of modest-to-severe energy deficiency, would improve immune function and physical performance. The carbohydrate delivery studies proposed by Dr. Zachwieja also could be important in the search for effective countermeasures.

Specific Comments, Concerns, and Questions for Tasks 5 and 8

The CMNR feels strongly that the advantages of using the human model for immunological studies far outweigh any advantages of using rat models. As noted earlier in this report, the rat models currently being developed for use in Tasks 3, 5, and 8 leave much to be desired in terms of their direct applicability to military situations involving stress. The use of a human model permits longer-term measurements of antibody response to test antigens as well as delayed dermal hypersensitivity responses. Also, immunological studies of rats can be impaired by lack of species-specific reagents. Both Drs. Zachwieja and Horohov have had extensive experience in conducting studies in human subjects. Combining Tasks 5 and 8 as human studies, and reducing the reliance on rodent studies, may have some economic advantages in the long run.

Recommendations for Tasks 5 and 8

The CMNR believes that the proposed new tasks, once the work being conducted within individual laboratory units becomes integrated and adapted to clinical and metabolic unit studies, will have high degrees of military relevance and should be supported as new areas of research.

Metabolic Unit Projects

Project Summary

An overview of the Metabolic Unit Projects was presented by Donna H. Ryan, M.D.; Jeffery J. Zachwieja, Ph.D.; and Steven R. Smith, M.D. During the past funding period, with input from the Army two metabolic studies were conducted. The first study, "Assessment of Intra- and Inter-Individual Metabolic Variation in Special Operations Forces Soldiers," sought to determine the possible need for individually-designed diets to optimize performance in Special Operations Forces soldiers, who are highly trained and severely stressed. The outcome of the study suggests that the inter-individual variation in response to changes in dietary carbohydrate is small and does not warrant individualization of military diets.

The second study, "Effects of Prolonged Inactivity on Musculoskeletal and Cardiovascular Systems with Evaluation of a Potential Countermeasure," reported by Dr. Smith, was done in conjunction with NASA and USARIEM. It sought to establish a rapidly developing model of microgravity that could then be used to test possible interventions for use by the space program. A model has been developed that involves administering low doses of tri-iodothyronine (T3) in conjunction with bed rest to mimic the effects of inactivity. After 4 weeks, changes in bone resorption markers are similar to those seen in more conventional human models after 4 months.

General Comments

The Metabolic Unit facility, in conjunction with the Stable Isotope Laboratory and Clinical Research Laboratory, provides an outstanding opportunity to control dietary interventions and physical conditions and to perform analyses of related metabolic parameters so that specific questions of interest to the military can be studied effectively. Future plans include testing interventions using testosterone and exercise. The CMNR is concerned with the use of female subjects in further investigations of the musculoskeletal response to microgravity. Until demonstrable countermeasures to maintain bone and muscle mass can be developed in males, female subjects should not be used because of their increased risk related to bone density.

The design of the physical facility and the equipment available for metabolic studies at the Pennington Biomedical Research Center are outstanding, and the available staff are well trained and experienced in the conduct of metabolic studies.

Specific Comments, Concerns, and Questions

No further use of the Metabolic Unit was proposed in the preproposal presented for this funding period. The rationale presented was that use of an animal model would be less expensive than experiments involving the Metabolic Unit. However, in listening to the proposals to evaluate work performance, diet, and immune function, the CMNR believes that much of the proposed work could be conducted better and with more direct application to the needs of the military using human subjects (see Tasks 5 and 8).

Recommendations

The CMNR recommends the use of human subjects in metabolic studies as these studies will be more inclusive and better directed to the needs of the military.

The CMNR recommends seeking the advice of additional experts in the field of bone mineral metabolism in the design and implementation of studies on microgravity, to maximize the efficacy of research while minimizing the risk to subjects. This area of research appears to be of greater importance for NASA than for the Army, and any further development and support should be provided by NASA.

SUMMARY OF THE COMMITTEE'S REVIEW

A summary of the scientific support services and related tasks, linking each task area outlined in the preproposal with its core laboratory support, as well as the recommendations of the CMNR, is provided in Table 1.

OVERALL CONCLUSIONS AND RECOMMENDATIONS

• The committee finds that the Clinical Research Laboratory is vital to the Pennington Biomedical Research Center and to the Military Nutrition Division at USARIEM. The availability of this laboratory to USARIEM has, in large measure, solved a critical need that existed for some time prior to 1990 to obtain timely and accurate analytical support for field studies on the nutritional status of military personnel and for the evaluation of military rations designed to meet their needs.

• Of concern to the committee is the lower than expected rate of publication in the scientific literature of the data produced for USARIEM by the Pennington Biomedical Research Center. The data acquired by this facility on energy requirements under a variety of circumstances (altitude exposure in men and women, extremes of physical training), changes in body composition with dietary and activity manipulations, and optimization of performance with dietary manipulations, would be of significant importance to the military as well as to the general scientific community. While the research may be reported in Army Technical Bulletins, the value of the work done by the PBRC in conjunction with USARIEM would be enhanced by publication in peer reviewed journals.

• The committee recommends continued support for and integration of the Clinical Research Laboratory, Stable Isotope Laboratory, Menu Modification/Enhancing Military Diets Project, and Nutrient Database Integration Laboratory at a level consistent with USARIEM needs. Experimental studies utilizing the technique of doubly labeled water as well as the incorporation of studies within the Metabolic Units Project employing isotopes to evaluate nutrient utilization should receive high priority in developing projects of interest to the Army.

• The committee recommends that additional collaborations be sought for the incorporation of the most current laboratory methodologies for nutrient analysis, with restriction of effort to obtaining data that are not currently available or extrapolative.

• The committee recommends that additional expenditure of resources be permitted for collaboration on and development and testing of various clinical laboratory tests to assess immune function.

• The committee recommends the use of human subjects in metabolic studies that will be more inclusive and better directed to the needs of the military.

• The committee believes that with expert consultation and with the development of an appropriate animal model to evaluate the impact of stress on brain function, the Stress, Nutrition, and Work Performance project can contribute much in the way of basic studies in support of the military mission. On the other hand, the committee does not feel that continuing the development

TABLE 1 Summary of Scientific Support Services, Related Tasks, and CMNR Recommendations

Laboratory/Facility	Current Task	Proposed Task	CMNR Recommendation
Clinical Nutrition Reference Laboratory (Task 1)	Clinical lab projects	Clinical lab projects	Continue development and support of clinical lab projects Integrate with Task 2 and Metabolic Unit Projects
Food Chemistry Laboratory	Menu Modification/Enhancing Military Diets Project (Task 6)	Menu Modification/Enhancing Military Diets Project (Task 6)	Promote further development and integration of Tasks 6 and 7
Nutrient Database Integration Laboratory (Task 7)	Nutrient Database Integration Laboratory (Task 7)	Nutrient Database Integration Laboratory (Task 7)	Promote further development and integration of Tasks 6 and 7
Stable Isotope Laboratory (Task 2)	Available as needed	Available as needed	Integrate Task 5 (Stress, Nutrition, and Work Performance, basic and clinical studies) and Task 8 (Stress, Nutrition, and Immune Function, basic and clinical studies) with these and Metabolic Unit Projects
Energy Expenditure/ Exercise Physiology Facilities	Available as needed	Available as needed	Continue stable isotope studies and integrate with Tasks 5 and 8 as well as Metabolic Unit Projects

TABLE 1 *Continued*

Laboratory/Facility	Current Task	Proposed Task	CMNR Recommendation
Body Composition Facilities	Available as needed	Available as needed	Continue stable isotope studies and integrate with Tasks 5 and 8 as well as Metabolic Unit Projects
Nutritional Neurosciences Laboratory	Stress, Nutrition, and Mental Performance (Task 3, basic studies)	Stress, Nutrition, and Mental Performance (Task 3, basic studies)	Continue Task 3 basic studies with modifications
Sleep Deprivation Laboratory	Stress, Sleep Deprivation, and Performance (Task 4, basic and clinical studies)	Stress, Sleep Deprivation, and Performance (Task 4, basic and clinical studies)	Discontinue clinical studies on sleep deprivation under Task 4
Stress, Nutrition, and Immune Function Laboratory		Stress, Nutrition, and Work Performance (Task 5, basic and clinical studies)	Integrate Tasks 5 and 8 for both basic and clinical studies with Metabolic Unit Projects
		Stress, Nutrition, and Immune Function (Task 8, basic and clinical studies)	

of clinical studies on sleep deprivation in the Sleep Laboratory is of particular value to the Army.

• The committee finds that the Menu Modification/Enhancing Military Diets Project as well as the Nutrient Database Integration Laboratory are valuable to the Army mission and provide needed support to USARIEM. Additional efforts with regard to nutrition education should be incorporated in order to meet Military Dietary Goals.

• The committee recommends integrating the proposed new projects, "Stress, Nutrition, and Work Performance" (Task 5) and "Stress, Nutrition and Immune Function" (Task 8), in both the basic laboratory studies and the clinical studies; they can provide a high degree of military relevance and should be strongly supported. Whenever possible and as appropriate, human subjects should be utilized rather than animal models in these project areas.

The CMNR is pleased to provide this review as part of the committee's continuing response to the U.S. Army Medical Research and Materiel Command. The committee always welcomes comments and suggestions regarding how these reports can better serve the needs of the Army.

ACKNOWLEDGMENTS

The CMNR expresses its appreciation to Donna H. Ryan, M.D., principal investigator for the military nutrition grant, and George A. Bray, M.D., director of the PBRC, for their hospitality during the site visit and the excellent organization of the review procedures and the background material provided prior to the visit. The committee thanks the PBRC scientists who presented summaries of their activities, proposed plans for the future, and patiently answered questions and were very forthcoming on requested information.

The CMNR chair wishes to acknowledge the excellent contribution of the FNB staff, especially Rebecca B. Costello, Ph.D., the project director of the CMNR, and Sydne J. Carlson-Newberry, Ph.D., staff officer of the CMNR, for the organization of the review and handling the many details necessary to prepare the report for publication. The comments by FNB director Allison A. Yates, Ph.D., provided helpful insights into the development of this final document. The chair also acknowledges the considerable skills of Susan M. Knasiak, research assistant, in assisting in the development of the review document, and Donna F. Allen, senior project assistant, for her work in making arrangements for the site visit. The excellent dedication of the entire FNB staff has made the desired fast reporting on this project review a reality.

Also, the chair continues to be extremely pleased with the dedication, cooperation, and excellence of the critical review that the members of the CMNR bring to this activity in support of the military nutrition research program. It is a real pleasure to work with such a cooperative, hard working, and friendly group.

REFERENCES

IOM (Institute of Medicine). 1992. A Nutritional Assessment of U.S. Army Ranger Training Class 11/91. A brief report of the Committee on Military Nutrition Research, Food and Nutrition Board. March 23, 1992. Washington, D.C.

IOM. 1993. Review of the Results of Nutritional Intervention, U.S. Army Ranger Training Class 11/92 (Ranger II), B.M. Marriott, ed. A report of the Committee on Military Nutrition Research, Food and Nutrition Board. Washington, D.C.: National Academy Press.

Appendix H

Conclusions and Recommendations from the Workshop Report Emerging Technologies for Nutrition Research

Submitted September 1997

Committee Responses to Questions, Conclusions, and Recommendations

As outlined in Chapter 1, the Committee on Military Nutrition Research (CMNR) was asked to provide a survey of newly available and emerging technologies that may be of significant value to the military for assessing and optimizing nutritional, physiological, and cognitive status and performance in military personnel. The following six categories of technologies were identified and evaluated for their applicability to the military mission:

- assessment of body composition,
- tracer techniques for study of metabolic processes,
- improved measures of energy expenditure and respiratory exchange,
- molecular and cellular approaches for evaluating nutritional requirements and status,
- assessment of immune status and function, and
- functional and behavioral measures of nutritional status.

The Military Nutrition Division (MND) (currently the Military Nutrition and Biochemical Division) at the U.S. Army Research Institute of Environmental Medicine (USARIEM) posed six questions for the CMNR to aid in its evaluation of the techniques reviewed and its provision of guidance to MND concerning their applications to the military.

In this chapter, the CMNR provides its answers to the questions posed by the Army, draws its conclusions on each of the six technologies reviewed, and makes its recommendations. The responses, conclusions, and recommendations were developed in discussion and prepared in executive session of the CMNR.

RESPONSES TO QUESTIONS POSED BY THE ARMY

This section is organized according to the six categories of technologies, with all of the Army's questions being answered under each technology.

Techniques of Body Composition Assessment

1. Will the technologies be a significant improvement over current technologies?

Anthropometric equations currently used by the military could be further refined with additional computer modeling, particularly with regard to their application to all ethnic groups. Computerized axial tomography (CAT) scanning, magnetic resonance imaging (MRI), and dual-energy x-ray absorptiometry (DXA) measurements can and have markedly improved compositional methodology in the clinic. These techniques could be used by the military to improve the accuracy and reliability of derived equations that use anthropometric measures to predict body fat content.

Single-frequency bioelectrical impedance analysis (BIA) is not a reliable measure of body composition, but the methodology may be helpful in answering specific questions concerning hydration status. Multiple-frequency bioelectrical impedance spectroscopy may hold promise for compositional measurement in the future.

2. How likely are the technologies to mature sufficiently for practical use?

Body composition (BC) methods are already quite mature, although multiple-frequency BIA requires some specific developmental work. The multifrequency method of BIA involves a simple and low-cost measurement system, but it is not sufficiently developed to provide accurate and reproducible estimates of changes in body composition. Its relative simplicity and low cost suggest that further development may be useful to see if current shortcomings can be overcome.

At present, CAT scanning, MRI, and DXA provide reliable measures of composition but are expensive. CAT requires exposure to x rays, although some CAT scanners have been modified to reduce x-ray exposure, so this may no longer be a limitation. While all these techniques lack ease of use in the field, DXA at least appears to have the potential to serve as a new criterion measure to validate anthropometric equations.

3. What is the cost/benefit ratio of the new technologies, and how expensive (in both monetary and personnel terms) will they be to employ compared with the importance of the information they will provide?

Anthropometric measurements and BIA are low cost and reasonably noninvasive (although a period of training is required to perform the former measurements accurately). The equipment required for CAT scanning, MRI, and DXA are high cost ($100,000–$1,000,000), and the training required to utilize the equipment is considerable. These costs, as well as the time required to perform the measurements on an individual, are a major limitation. Therefore, these techniques have value primarily as research tools (criterion measures) to aid in refining practical anthropometric methods for everyday use.

4. Are the technologies of such critical value that their development should be supported by Department of Defense (DoD) funds—such as can be provided by the Small Business Innovative Research (SBIR) program?

Because fat-free mass (FFM) is the only BC component that appears to be correlated with physical performance capacity, technology is needed for the accurate estimation of muscle mass, lean body mass, or FFM.

To assess the effects of military operations on body composition in individual soldiers, improvement is needed in methods for assessment and prediction of modest longitudinal changes in body composition. While DXA might provide the most accurate, direct longitudinal assessment, its relatively limited practicality in the field makes it a more likely candidate to be the criterion against which new anthropometric equations can be validated.

Research with CAT, MRI, and DXA will continue in the private sector because of the medical applications of these technologies, including their potential to assess changes in body composition.

Multifrequency BIA represents a simple technology that, if it could be developed sufficiently to overcome its current shortcomings, may be a technology whose adaptation for military field use could benefit from additional development funding. Anthropometric measurements may need additional support from computer development in the refinement of predictive equations. Such fine tuning of anthropometric methods is low cost and would likely be performed in-house or with limited outside support.

5. **How practical are the technologies? Will they require dedicated personnel and complex, exotic equipment? Will the data provided be difficult to analyze?**

Anthropometric measurements and BIA are practical, although trained technicians should be utilized to perform these measurements. The large scanning devices are best used for developing predictive equations although mobile units are available. Cooperative work with medical or other institutions to utilize existing facilities and trained personnel appears to be the most practical and economical approach, as such facilities are experienced in collecting and analyzing data from these devices.

6. **Can the technologies be used in the field (could they be used in the field or used to analyze samples collected in the field)?**

Anthropometric measurements can be conducted in the field. Although BIA also can be performed in the field, it currently does not represent an improvement over anthropometric measures of BC. Because the interpretation of BIA predictions of body composition is influenced significantly by environmental factors, health status, and physical activity, its use in the field may provide a mechanism for easily monitoring these factors, which are of significant interest to the military. Although mobile units are available for DXA and MRI, their use in the field to measure small changes in body composition is costly in terms of technician time. Hence, the use of these latter instruments is limited to validation of currently used anthropometric equations.

Tracer Techniques for the Study of Metabolism

1. **Will the technologies be a significant improvement over current technologies?**

Major advances in the understanding and measurement of metabolic processes have been made by incorporating these methodologies into studies of substrate utilization, energy requirements, and muscle function. The methods provide a safe mechanism for monitoring metabolites that was not available previously.

2. **How likely are the technologies to mature sufficiently for practical use?**

Tracer methodology is developed and mature, although new labels, new techniques for separation of labeled metabolites (mass isotopomer distribution analysis), and more sensitive spectrometers are increasing its application. The doubly labeled water (DLW) technique has been used in field studies to estimate energy expenditure in troops. Other isotopic procedures have been used in laboratory settings to evaluate fuel use during exercise, and nuclear magnetic resonance (NMR) has been developed to assess intracellular metabolites and fuel stores. Reliable and reproducible data are best provided by laboratory groups with significant experience in the measurement and interpretation of the data obtained.

3. What is the cost/benefit ratio of the new technologies, and how expensive (in both monetary and personnel terms) will they be to employ compared with the importance of the information they will provide?

Compounds labeled with stable isotopes are moderately expensive and the mass spectrometers required for analysis are expensive ($100,000–$300,000), but the cost of such measurements can be reduced with batch processing of labeled compounds and the use of core facilities. There is significant variation in the cost of studies utilizing this technology.

When tracer isotopes can be administered and samples collected noninvasively in the field, cost is minimized. Samples and data can be analyzed in a core laboratory, and costs can be kept at a relatively low level for the value of the data obtained (an example being DLW studies of energy expenditure of troops in field operations). Incorporation of NMR or positron emission tomography (PET) greatly increases study expenses.

When invasive techniques are required for administration and collection of samples, the stable isotope methods described are largely confined to laboratory use. However, for the information obtained using these stable isotope methods, the amount of data acquired is immense.

NMR carries a large initial outlay for the magnet and the physicist to run it, but individual measurements are inexpensive to make, and the noninvasive nature increases its appeal.

PET is prohibitively expensive ($2,000,000), and its use is limited to those facilities where sufficient medical need warrants its purchase. The information on metabolic processes that can be derived from this method is, as yet, untapped.

4. Are the technologies of such critical value that their development should be supported by DoD funds—such as can be provided by the SBIR program?

The use of these techniques has developed in medical, nutrition, and physiology laboratories to improve the understanding of metabolic processes. It is a very active research field, heavily supported by federal funding. The MND should keep abreast of developments in the field to identify areas where the application to military nutrition is important. Funding for projects of specific interest to the military may be considered, but general funding is not necessary for this technology to develop rapidly.

5. How practical are the technologies? Will they require dedicated personnel and complex, exotic equipment? Will the data provided be difficult to analyze?

Studies using stable isotopes require trained personnel for design and implementation. The technique is not trivial, nor is data analysis, so that experienced personnel are required to ensure meaningful results. Within that framework, the ease of the technique depends on the mode of dosing and sampling. Oral dosing followed by urine sampling is practical and easy for subjects. Intravenous dosing and arterial sampling require medical personnel and facilities.

NMR and PET require little on the part of the subject, but highly trained personnel must run the equipment.

6. Can the technologies be used in the field (could they be used in the field or used to analyze samples collected in the field)?

Studies involving invasive procedures to deliver isotope and collect samples are inappropriate for field work at this time. Studies that require magnets or cyclotrons cannot be performed easily in the field at this time.

Ambulatory Techniques for Measurement of Energy Expenditure

1. Will the technologies be a significant improvement over current technologies?

The DLW technique is a major improvement over the use of portable indirect calorimetry for estimating energy expenditure in the field. However, the use of ambulatory monitoring devices is an evolving technology that shows promise for use in estimating energy expenditure in the field as well.

The application of near-infrared (NIR) spectroscopy, if perfected, could permit the noninvasive measurement of plasma metabolites, such as glucose, using a portable instrument with the accuracy and reliability of currently used blood-based methods. The difficulty in differentiating multiple metabolites in blood only may be overcome slowly.

2. How likely are the technologies to mature sufficiently for practical use?

The measurement of total energy expenditure with doubly labeled water is already practical for field use. Activity monitoring remains a fertile field of investigation as newer methods of measuring activity and energy expenditure are integrated.

NIR spectroscopy techniques and instrumentation are currently in use for routine food analysis and for blood flow monitoring of tissue oxygenation and are well developed. The measurement of a broad variety of other plasma metabolites, such as blood glucose, is an emerging technology that is not yet fully developed. Blood is a complex mixture of many organic compounds, each with overlapping spectra in the NIR range. In addition, blood flow is dynamic, and many plasma metabolites are in constant flux, particularly under conditions of stress. These represent formidable methodological obstacles not yet overcome, either by transcutaneous or reflectance NIR measurements. An additional obstacle is the unavailability, to date, of the portable equipment that would be required for field use. This is an area of considerable investigation.

3. What is the cost/benefit ratio of the new technologies, and how expensive (in both monetary and personnel terms) will they be to employ compared with the importance of the information they will provide?

Doubly labeled water carries a fairly high price tag due to the costs of isotope (about \$400–\$500 per dose) and analysis (about \$500 per dose). This cost is somewhat balanced by the ease of use, quantity of data produced, and safety of subjects. Portable oxygen consumption devices and ambulatory monitors are reasonably inexpensive and easy for subjects to use.

Although the equipment that is required for portable, noninvasive testing of plasma metabolites using NIR spectroscopy would be relatively inexpensive to build and operate, the cost of development of that equipment could be great.

4. Are the technologies of such critical value that their development should be supported by DoD funds—such as can be provided by the SBIR program?

The use of stable isotopes to measure energy expenditure is a well-developed method that requires no further support for development. Funds should continue to be appropriated to support the development of ambulatory monitoring, to refine the technology under development, and to validate the devices with field studies. The "foot strike" method is interesting and may be more useful if it can be applied to uneven terrain. This method is less expensive than isotopic methods and could be applied readily to significant numbers of individuals in the field.

The large potential market in the civilian sector for noninvasive, portable medical devices employing NIR spectroscopy for the measure of plasma metabolites should drive the development of suitable instrumentation. No investment should be required on the part of the military.

5. How practical are the technologies? Will they require dedicated personnel and complex, exotic equipment? Will the data provided be difficult to analyze?

The DLW method for determination of energy expenditure is fairly practical to administer in the field, although interpretation is complicated by changes in water supply and large changes in activity patterns. Thus, analysis is sometimes problematic, and sample handling and data interpretation require trained personnel.

Measures of oxygen consumption or ambulatory monitors are used more easily by individuals in the field but need further field testing. The data obtained are readily interpretable by computer analysis, but personnel who perform that interpretation require some training.

Noninvasive field applications of NIR spectroscopy will require simple, rugged, and portable equipment, while routine health screening of military personnel at their home bases would have less stringent equipment requirements. However, at the present time, neither the technology nor the necessary instrumentation are available for either of these applications.

6. Can the technologies be used in the field (could they be used in the field or used to analyze samples collected in the field)?

The performance of studies on energy expenditure in the field has a long history. The DLW technique has been widely used in the field and has yielded useful information in a variety of military studies. Studies of energy expenditure employing the DLW technique require oral dosing and urine sampling, and at present such studies are routinely conducted in the field; however, this method has only limited applicability due to cost. The foot strike method will benefit from more development and evaluation in a variety of field applications.

When simple, rugged, and portable NIR spectroscopy equipment is developed to measure blood flow, tissue oxygen saturation, and a variety of plasma metabolites, it is possible to see many important field applications both in training and in other operations.

Molecular and Cellular Approaches to Nutrition

1. Will the technologies be a significant improvement over current technologies?

At the present time, the use of molecular cloning techniques to elucidate the human genome, study the control of gene expression, and control the synthesis of particular desirable or undesirable gene products both *in vivo* and *in vitro* is rapidly advancing the front and the pace of research in many areas. The techniques described represent the state of the art for most applications of molecular biology and are widely used in both academic and industrial research laboratories.

In many respects, the use of isolated cell systems represents a significant advance over other methods (tissue culture and perfused organ systems, for example) for the study of cellular responses to external stimuli. The techniques await validation against appropriate *in vivo* measurements to demonstrate their true potential.

2. How likely are the technologies to mature sufficiently for practical use?

Apart from the use of molecular cloning techniques to facilitate *in vitro* production of cellular products, such as vaccines, and improve the food supply, the most promising application for these technologies at the present time and in the near future is basic research. By bringing the investigation down to the level of gene expression, it is becoming possible to elucidate completely the mechanisms, by which stimuli, such as environmental stresses or changes in nutritional status, exert their influence upon physiological systems.

Isolated cell techniques will find practical use largely, if not solely, in basic research settings. The likelihood that they will yield valid or useful information will depend on the effort that is expended to choose an appropriate model system and validate it properly. With the exception of the use of red cell hemolysis to assess vitamin E status, the use of isolated cells for determination of nutritional status is not an available technology at this time.

3. What is the cost/benefit ratio of the new technologies, and how expensive (in both monetary and personnel terms) will they be to employ compared with the importance of the information they will provide?

These are technical approaches that at the present time are almost exclusively limited in their application to the basic research setting. They require a considerable investment of capital for equipment and materials, time, and personnel to develop a well-conceived research plan. While the information obtained by the use of molecular cloning techniques could not be obtained in any other way, the potential benefit of obtaining such information must be evaluated by anyone considering undertaking such research.

Isolated cell approaches, in contrast, may be comparable in cost to molecular cloning techniques, yet the value of the information they can provide largely remains to be demonstrated (even within the scientific community).

4. Are the technologies of such critical value that their development should be supported by DoD funds—such as can be provided by the SBIR program?

This technology is under active investigation in a variety of settings and supported by federal and private industry funding. Unless a specific application to a military setting is recognized, the CMNR does not recommend DoD funding at this time. At some point, as the technology develops, DoD may wish to evaluate whether its support would help a specific area, such as the effect of oxidative stress on gene expression, in view of the number of military settings where oxidative stress may be of particular concern.

5. How practical are the technologies? Will they require dedicated personnel and complex, exotic equipment? Will the data provided be difficult to analyze?

At this time, techniques of molecular biology are not practical to answer nutritional questions of military significance. This type of work demands a considerable amount of equipment (although it is equipment that is currently available), extensive training, and the knowledge base to analyze the data. In addition, the development of the testing protocols alone for any product that emerges as a result of research conducted at the molecular biology level will require that a number of ethical and safety questions be taken into consideration.

If isolated cell techniques can be validated sufficiently, it is conceivable that they might be utilized to study samples drawn from individuals working in the field and transported to a laboratory in a remote location.

6. Can the technologies be used in the field (could they be used in the field or used to analyze samples collected in the field)?

While there is no reason to imagine conducting basic molecular biological or cell physiology research in the field, several field applications may become feasible in the future. One application that will become more appealing as the elucidation of the human genome progresses is the screening of cells taken from individuals recently exposed to extreme environmental conditions (stimuli) to determine the effects of these stimuli on gene expression. Such testing could be accomplished by sampling the tissues or cells of interest (if it can be done non-invasively) in the field setting and transporting them to a remote laboratory. Similar studies could be done to elucidate subcellular physiological processes using isolated cell approaches. A second application would involve techniques of gene transfer. These techniques, which are just now being developed and tested in humans who have been diagnosed with any of several rare genetic disorders or terminal cancers, may impart the ability to synthesize proteins not otherwise made by the body because of a missing or defective gene or some alteration in the regulatory process. The potential clearly exists to enhance the expression of particular genes or to place their expression under the control of nutrients (such as zinc) or some other dietary or environmental stimulus. Procedures of this sort await extensive testing, not to mention the solution of a myriad of ethical and practical questions, before realistic field applications can be considered.

Assessment of Immune Function

1. Will the technologies be a significant improvement over current technologies?

Improved methodologies for measuring functions of cell-mediated immunity and cytokine production are extensions of current methodologies. These generally are available in academic research institutions.

Novel approaches to the development of oral vaccines for active immunizations, and human antibodies for passive immunization, represent vastly important improvements over current technologies and give great promise for inducing better and more complete immunity than do current vaccines, and at a far lower cost.

2. How likely are the technologies to mature sufficiently for practical use?

Testing methodologies for evaluating immune system functions are constantly being studied and improved in academic centers. Whenever available, these improved methods will need to be adapted by military laboratories and modified for field use.

Exciting new methodologies and approaches for the development of oral vaccines are being pursued vigorously by many groups, and the first human testing of experimental new vaccines should occur shortly. Since the Army is already highly engaged in the development of uniquely important military vaccines, new technologies for vaccine development are of great potential importance.

The possible creation of specific, human-compatible antibodies by the development and use of transgenic plants represents an important medical advance which could be of great value to military medicine. Such antibodies could be used to confer weeks to months of prophylactic passive immunity, or they could be used as specific forms of therapy. The transgenic antibodies would replace and expand the diversity of the available and costly passive immunization practices, which require the gathering and processing of human serum or the much more dangerous use of serum obtained form horses or other animals.

3. What is the cost/benefit ratio of the new technologies, and how expensive (in both monetary and personnel terms) will they be to employ compared with the importance of the information they will provide?

The testing of immunological functions tends to be quite expensive, especially when these tests can only be done in research laboratories using costly reagents and equipment. Costs for field testing could be minimized (in terms of both money and loss of duty time by military personnel) if immunological studies could be limited to specific tests that prove to be most meaningful and reliable.

Tests based on cytokine assays, especially those of the proinflammatory cytokines and related molecules excreted in urine, have great potential for adding important new diagnostic measures at a relatively inexpensive cost/benefit ratio.

Costs of developing and testing potential new oral vaccines are likely to be comparable with those of conventional vaccines currently under development. However, oral vaccines have the potential for being far cheaper to produce (especially if effective antigens or antibodies can be produced in transgenic plants), and for being safer, more effective, and less costly to administer.

4. Are the technologies of such critical value that their development should be supported by DoD funds—such as can be provided by the SBIR program?

The occurrence of immune system dysfunctions, such as those induced by one episode of Ranger training and those that may arise in the course of basic combat training or any military operation, needs to be investigated further. Such investigations should be extended to other operational situations that involve extreme physical stress and weight loss. In conducting these investigations, the DoD should employ the best available testing methodologies and adapt them to field use whenever necessary.

Infectious diseases continue to have high DoD costs in terms of both medical care and lost time for military personnel. Infection-induced losses of body weight and essential nutrients can then impair physical performance for long periods of time. DoD use of immunizations to prevent (or minimize) the military impact of infectious diseases (including those due to biological warfare threat agents) has included the need for DoD funding and in-house research to develop, test, and procure all unique vaccines of military importance that are not available commercially. The potential for developing new families of oral vaccines that are more effective, less expensive, and easier to administer than currently available vaccines should not be ignored by the DoD. Creation of new families of transgenic plant-produced antibodies for passive protection against rare infections and toxemias of potential military importance represents a technological breakthrough that should be developed fully by the DoD in the immediate future. The CMNR supports the recommendation that a Science and Technology Objective be established for adaptation of militarily relevant vaccines for oral administration, and transgenic antibodies for passive protection, through the application of new technologies described in this report.

5. How practical are the technologies? Will they require dedicated personnel and complex, exotic equipment? Will the data provided be difficult to analyze?

Advanced methodologies for a wide assortment of immunological assessments are already available in research laboratories, but considerable effort may be required to adapt them for field use. This problem can be minimized by focusing on a small, select number of tests that will yield the greatest amount of clinical information.

Methodologies for developing a variety of effective new oral vaccines have already proven to be highly practical, and the first of such experimental vaccines are becoming available for human testing. Development and testing of new vaccines of unique military importance will still require time and money. The same is true for development of human antibodies in transgenic plants.

6. Can the technologies be used in the field (could they be used in the field or used to analyze samples collected in the field)?

Field studies of Rangers in training have helped to highlight the immune dysfunctions that may be a consequence of these types of extreme environmental stress. Further such studies are needed to elucidate the nature and course of these immune system dysfunctions. Measurements of proinflammatory cytokines (such as IL-6 and IL-6 receptor antagonists) may be performed on single urine specimens collected in the field, although caution must be exercised in the interpretation of results. Further development of noninvasive assays (i.e., those that would use saliva, urine, stool, or other available samples), as well as simple, rugged, portable equipment for analyzing plasma metabolites and blood cell counts, should increase the ease of performing field measurements.

Immunization is an important component of preparation for battlefield readiness. Refinement of vaccine production and improvement of delivery systems will greatly assist in increasing the effectiveness of, and compliance with, immunization programs.

FUNCTIONAL AND BEHAVIORAL MEASURES OF NUTRITIONAL STATUS

1. Will the technologies be a significant improvement over current technologies?

These methods actually constitute a group of technologies that measure different aspects of physical and cognitive performance. For one of these techniques, Muscle Function Analysis (MFA), the basic premises underlying the association between collected data and lean body mass or other indicators of nutritional status remains to be validated. The effects of prior strenuous physical exercise on MFA readings are not clear nor is it possible as yet to eliminate the contribution of voluntary muscle contraction or changes in activity of the sodium potassium pump. Furthermore, although the MFA procedure is relatively noninvasive, it is considered painful. This technique has the advantage of providing data in a very short time.

Most of the methods of cognitive function assessment discussed in Chapters 24 and 25 represent the current state of the art. Some suggestions for new technologies, both those that were described in the chapters and those discussed during committee deliberations, were also considered. When miniaturization and interfaces are enhanced and portability is improved, such measures should have more field-relevant benefits for the military.

2. How likely are the technologies to mature sufficiently for practical use?

It is believed that within the next 5 years, studies validating the use of MFA for assessment of nutritional status should be completed and documented in the peer-reviewed literature. The device currently is being tested in healthy individuals, trauma patients, hemodialysis patients, HIV+ patients, and nutritionally compromised individuals in general hospital wards, both before and after realimentation. In subjects studied to date, contractile characteristics of healthy volunteers appear reliable, and the test appears to be capable of measuring rapid changes in nutritionally compromised patients following the initiation of refeeding.

Most of the cognitive assessment technologies discussed are already available. The inclusion of the ability to monitor or test cognitive function by incorporation of new technologies into existing equipment used by military personnel would be a significant step in nonintrusive testing. Such technologies should be readily available within 5 years, as required equipment is essentially available. Miniaturization may be required but should easily be developed.

3. What is the cost/benefit ratio of the new technologies, and how expensive (in both monetary and personnel terms) will they be to employ compared with the importance of the information they will provide?

The MFA apparatus is relatively inexpensive, as is the cost for use. Skilled technicians are required to perform the measurements. With proper validation, the cost/benefit ratio for this technique would be quite low, although personnel must leave their assigned tasks to be tested.

Some cognitive assessments, such as paper and pencil tests, are inexpensive but take personnel away from assigned tasks for short periods of time. Others, such as measures involving extensive computer hardware, other hardware (e.g., electroencephalogram monitors), or software programming have high start-up costs for equipment but are designed to monitor, rather than to interfere with, the functions and operations of personnel. The information gathered could be valuable for assessing the role of nutritional and other factors, such as sleep in the field. The use of devices such as simulators involves expensive equipment and also takes personnel away from their tasks to complete the tests.

4. Are the technologies of such critical value that their development should be supported by DoD funds—such as can be provided by the SBIR program?

Developments in the private sector need to be closely monitored by the DoD so that it may adapt what is already commercially available. Because most of the technologies are already developed, specific military field applications that involve miniaturization and increased portability should be financed by DoD.

5. How practical are the technologies? Will they require dedicated personnel and complex, exotic equipment? Will the data provided be difficult to analyze?

The practicality of the MFA device is problematic at present. Constant monitoring does not appear to be possible at this time. In addition, subjects must interrupt their tasks to be measured. Although the device is light enough to be transported to the field, it is somewhat cumbersome for continuous wear and restricts arm movement. Nevertheless, the measurement is noninvasive and inexpensive. The total measurement time is only 10 to 15 minutes, results are available immediately, and in the future, continuous monitoring may be possible.

The cognitive assessment technologies are already in use. Dedicated personnel needs are minimal except for data interpretation. The equipment is not complex or exotic, and most of it is already available. Analysis of these types of data has a long history, and few problems are anticipated; however, as with the MFA and many other assessment tools, personnel must leave their assigned tasks to participate in most tests of cognitive function.

6. Can the technologies be used in the field (could they be used in the field or used to analyze samples collected in the field)?

At present, the potential for use of MFA in the field appears to be low. Although the device is light and relatively portable, the validity of the technique remains to be demonstrated, and its use is associated with causing significant pain to the subject. Field use should be reevaluated in the future after existing problems are overcome.

The cognitive assessment techniques, with the exception of field simulators, are all applicable to field-testing scenarios. They await further improvements in miniaturization, portability, and durability.

COMMITTEE CONCLUSIONS

These conclusions were developed in executive session and represent the views of the CMNR.

• Methods of measuring body composition are relevant and important to the military to assure accuracy and fairness in the application of body composition measures to accession and retention of military personnel.

• Anthropometric measures are the most applicable methods for evaluating compliance with military standards of body fat. The more sophisticated technologies of CAT scanning, MRI, and DXA are useful tools for developing application equations from anthropometric measures to estimate body fat.

• BIA is a less-reliable method of measuring body fat at this time, but the methodology may be useful in answering specific questions concerning hydration state and function of cell membranes.

• Tracer methodology, particularly the use of stable isotopes, is an important technology for understanding and measuring metabolic processes (the doubly labeled water technique currently is used in studies of energy expenditure in the field and is a cost-effective technology for this purpose). Stable isotopes that can be administered and measured noninvasively through easily obtained samples offer important opportunities to estimate metabolic processes in the field. Central analysis of samples increases the practicality of their use in field studies.

• Ambulatory monitoring techniques, such as the foot strike measurement, also show good promise as field measures of work and energy expenditure.

• The various molecular and cellular technologies are interesting as research methods but are strictly laboratory research tools at present. Observing the development of these techniques and their application will be important for the MND at USARIEM, but investing in their in-house development is not recommended at this time. As questions develop that may be studied using these techniques, the DoD may wish to consider support for extramural research (for example, the effect of oxidative stress or malnutrition on gene expression).

• Studies of immune function are potentially very important to the military. An understanding of the effect of the various stresses of military operations on the body's immune function and how these may be modified to aid soldier performance is an important area for investigation.

• The development of vaccines that are effective against various infectious diseases of unique significance to the military population but not necessarily of significance to the civilian population may be very important in sustaining the ability of the soldier to operate effectively in the field. Oral vaccines may be most effective as they tend to mimic the route of exposure to the infectious agents that cause problems in the field.

• The development and production of human antibodies by transgenic plants create dramatic new possibilities for short-term (weeks-to-months) prophylaxis, or therapy, of unusual infectious diseases or toxemias of potential military importance and for which no other forms of immunization currently are available.

• The ability to study the cognitive performance of individuals while they perform their duties has great potential for improving soldier performance under stress. Current developments in computerized and miniaturized technology appear to permit expanded studies of real-time cognitive behavior. Support for the development of specific monitoring devices that are compatible with field military equipment may be necessary to implement this technology.

COMMITTEE RECOMMENDATIONS

The following recommendations are based on the CMNR's review and evaluation of the workshop discussions.

• Fair and equitable implementation of body fat and BMI standards is important to the military. It is recommended that continued research be carried out to refine the anthropometric measures using the sophisticated measurements of body composition provided by DXA, MRI, and/or CAT scanning to assure that measures used to evaluate personnel are equitable for gender, ethnic, and body type characteristics.

• The development and use of scanning technologies for the measurement of changes in body composition (particularly changes in muscle mass) that may result from field exercises should be refined in controlled laboratory environments and in collaboration with the civilian sector.

• Currently, multifrequency BIA is not sufficiently precise to be a useful tool for body composition determination. However, its potential as a simple field measure of hydrational status suggests that research to improve its value should be encouraged.

• Research by the private sector on the use of stable isotopes should be carefully monitored so that issues of concern to the military that can be studied effectively by these methods may be identified and the technology applied to the military situation when the costs versus the benefits are favorable. Since the effective application of this technology requires well-trained personnel and expensive and sophisticated equipment, the collaboration with other government and private sector laboratories in these studies continues to appear most expedient. In addition, as much information as possible should be obtained in well-controlled laboratory environments.

• The various molecular and cellular techniques for the study of nutrition and other physiological processes are strictly laboratory research tools at present and are not ready for implementation by the MND. Military problems that would appear to be amenable to investigation with these tools are of sufficiently broad interest as to be under consideration by established private-sector research laboratories. Maintaining awareness of the activities of these laboratories now receiving significant support by federal and industrial funds should continue, and therefore, DoD investment is not recommended at this time.

• Since military operations are frequently stressful and may be carried out in very hostile environments, it is important to understand the role that the body's immune function plays in helping the soldier cope and to consider ways in which immune responses may be controlled or enhanced to maximize the individual's ability to perform. Awareness of this research field and investment in selected research of potential significance to the military mission should be continued. The military must keep apprised of research findings on the influence of nutritional status on immune function.

• Research on possible vaccine programs that may protect soldiers from infectious diseases frequently encountered in military operations should be supported, particularly when the potential infections are not usually a problem in the civilian sector. Oral vaccine development should be encouraged. Preliminary research at U.S. Army Medical Research Institute for Infectious Diseases to develop militarily important oral vaccines should be expanded. Research should be initiated or funded to develop transgenic plants that can produce antibodies against infections or toxins of unique military importance and to assess the influence of nutritional status on the response of military personnel to vaccinations.

• The development of techniques and equipment that would permit evaluation of cognitive performance of individuals while actually performing their operational tasks should be supported, with the caveat that such techniques must be validated and as much information gathered as possible in controlled laboratory environments prior to field testing. When special modification is required for use in military equipment, support should be given to such development (for example, miniaturization).

The Committee on Military Nutrition Research is pleased to have participated with the Military Nutrition Division (currently the Military Nutrition and Biochemical Division), U.S. Army Research Institute of Environmental Medicine, and the U.S. Army Medical Research and Materiel Command in progress relating to the nutrition, performance, and health of U.S. military personnel. The CMNR hopes that this information will be valuable to the U.S. Department of Defense in developing programs that continue to improve the performance and lifelong health and well-being of service personnel.

Appendix I

Conclusions and Recommendations from the Workshop Report Assessing Readiness in Military Women

Submitted March 1998

Subcommittee Responses to Questions, Conclusions, and Recommendations

As outlined in Chapter 1, military personnel are required to adhere to standards of body composition, fitness, and appearance for the purpose of achieving and maintaining readiness. The purpose of this report is to examine whether the present standards for body composition, fitness, and appearance support readiness by ensuring optimal health and performance of active-duty women. After reviewing the relevant literature and current military policies, the Subcommittee on Body Composition, Nutrition, and Health provides the following conclusions and recommendations in response to the three questions posed by the military. Recommendations for future research are provided following the responses to the questions.

1. What body composition standards best serve military women's health and fitness, with respect to minimum lean body mass, maximum body fat, and site specificity of fat deposition? Are the appearance goals of the military in conflict with military readiness?

• The BCNH subcommittee recommends the revision of the two-tiered body composition and fitness screen.

As illustrated in Figure 1, the first tier should consist of semiannual assessment of BMI and fitness (including strength and endurance). The acceptable range of BMIs, based on considerations of health, is recommended to be 19 to 25, independent of age. Individuals whose BMI falls within the desirable range and who pass the fitness test need no further screening. Individuals with a BMI greater than 25 should be subjected to a second tier of screening, based on body fat assessment. The subcommittee believes that women with BMIs less than 19 can be fit to perform. However, as BMI decreases below 19, women may be at risk for malnutrition and should be considered for medical evaluation.

Individuals whose body fat is assessed at 36 percent or less and who pass the fitness test will be considered within standard. Individuals whose body fat exceeds 30 percent and who fail the fitness test will be referred to weight management and fitness programs. Individuals whose body fat exceeds 36 percent will be referred to a weight management program, regardless of fitness score.

• The BCNH subcommittee also recommends development of a single service-wide equation derived from circumference measurements for assessment of women's body fat, to be validated against a four-compartment model using a population of active-duty women or a population that is identical in ethnic and

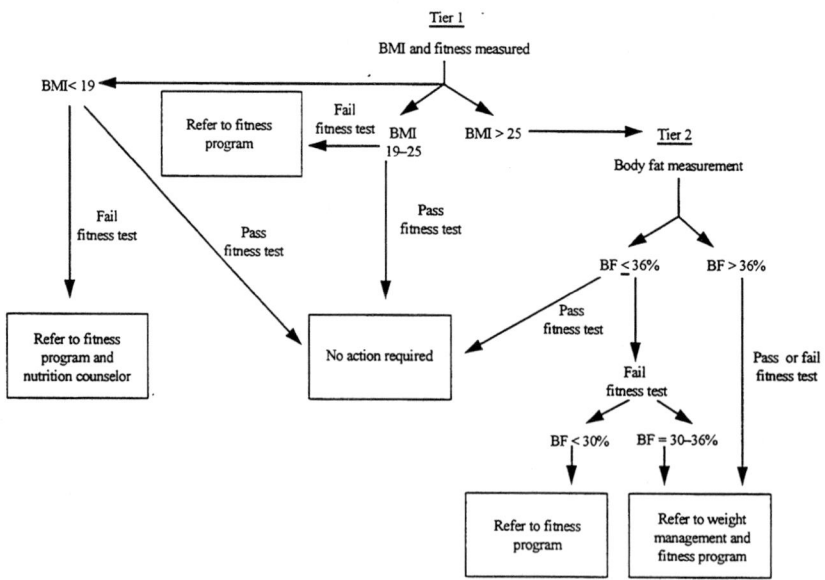

FIGURE 1 Revised flow chart for screening recommendation. BMI, body mass index; BF, body fat.

age diversity to that of military women. Development and validation of this equation may result in reconsideration of the recommended BMI cut-offs, in part as a result of establishing the measurement error.

• The BCNH subcommittee recommends an increasing emphasis on general fitness for health and readiness by enforcing uniformly across all services and MOSs regular and monitored participation in a fitness program consisting of a minimum of 3 d/wk of endurance exercise at 60 to 80 percent of maximum capacity for 20 to 60 minutes and 2 d/wk of resistance exercise using all major muscle groups at 85 percent of one repetition maximum (ACSM, 1990). Such a program, in addition to promoting fitness, assists in maintenance of weight and FFM and may result in lower body fat. Periodic fitness and body composition testing adjusted appropriately for gender should be conducted to determine both endurance and strength and should be similar across all services. More frequent testing would promote continuous adherence to weight and physical fitness programs and decrease injurious behaviors that result from efforts to pass performance and body composition tests.

• The subcommittee further recommends development of task-specific, gender-neutral strength and endurance tests and standards for use in the determination of placement in MOSs that require moderate and heavy lifting. Additional fitness programs should be created and enforced to develop and maintain the strength, endurance, and flexibility required by these MOSs.

• The BCNH subcommittee recommends that, in view of the association between FFM (as an indirect indicator of skeletal muscle mass) and strength, the military consider developing an appropriate minimum recommended BMI for accession of women.

• The current appearance standard does not appear to be linked to performance, fitness, nutrition, or health. The BCNH subcommittee recommends that if the military deems appearance standards to be necessary, objective criteria (that do not discriminate on the basis of ethnicity) should be developed and utilized.

2. Should any part of the MRDAs be further adjusted for women? Should there be any intervention for active-duty women with respect to food provided, dietary supplementation, or education?

• In view of current ongoing efforts by the Food and Nutrition Board to revise the RDAs upon which the MRDAs (AR 40-25, 1985) are based, the BCNH subcommittee advises that revision of the MRDAs be deferred to a later time and has chosen to concentrate on several nutritional issues of importance to active-duty women.

• The BCNH subcommittee reinforces the requirement for adequate energy and nutrient intakes to reflect the needs of the body at a moderate activity level

(2,000–2,800 kcal/d). To ensure adequate nutrient intakes, female personnel must be educated on how to meet both energy and nutrient needs whether they are deployed and subsisting on operational rations or whether they are in garrison. This education is required to enable women to choose foods of higher nutrient density and to maintain a fitness program that will allow greater energy intake. The subcommittee reinforces the recent efforts of the Army to begin providing complete nutritional labeling of all ration components and to include information to enable identification of nutrient-dense components that would help women meet the MRDAs at their usual energy intake. The subcommittee also supports efforts to create ration supplements that would satisfy requirements that may not be readily met through the usual intake of rations. The subcommittee recommends nutritional labeling of all dining hall menu items and provision of food selection guidelines to women in garrison.

• The BCNH subcommittee recommends that all military women maintain or achieve healthy weight through a continuous exercise and fitness program. If weight loss is a goal, nutrition education and ongoing counseling should be provided for guidance in achieving a healthy, but reduced energy, diet. Emphasis must be placed on preventing overweight and maintaining long-term weight management through lifestyle changes, rather than on crash dieting to lose weight for a scheduled weigh-in. Adequate energy intake should be encouraged to reduce risks of injury and amenorrhea.

3. What special guidance should be offered with respect to return-to-duty standards and nutrition for women who are pregnant or breastfeeding?

• The BCNH subcommittee recommends that all women be encouraged to eat an adequate diet during pregnancy and lactation as recommended by the IOM (1990, 1991). The subcommittee further recommends an intake of 400 µg/d dietary folate during childbearing years, 600 µg/d dietary folate during pregnancy and 500 µg/d during lactation as recommended by the IOM (1998). A daily supplement of 30 mg of ferrous iron (IOM, 1990) is recommended during the second and third trimesters of pregnancy. During pregnancy and lactation, women should abstain from smoking. Although alcohol should be avoided during pregnancy, a very moderate intake may be permitted during lactation (IOM, 1990).

• The BCNH subcommittee recommends that pregnant women without obstetrical or medical complications engage in moderate levels of physical activity to maintain cardiovascular and muscular fitness throughout the pregnancy and the postpartum period. The American College of Obstetricians and Gynecologists (ACOG, 1994) has published guidelines that should be used to advise pregnant active-duty women to modify their physical fitness program. Programs should be individualized and made available to healthy women who can and wish to exercise. These programs may also incorporate strength training, although the extent of the benefits of such training during pregnancy remains to be determined.

• The BCNH subcommittee recommends the endorsement of the IOM guidelines for gestational weight gain as outlined in the text. Women should be encouraged to gain within the IOM recommendations during pregnancy and to lose weight postpartum through appropriate nutritional counseling and exercise programs. The BCNH subcommittee recommends that the proposed time allowance for compliance to weight and body fat standards postpartum be consistent with IOM recommendations for gestational weight gain. When satisfactory progress is being made toward compliance, an allowance of up to 1 year postpartum should be given for attainment of body weight standards.

• Resumption of exercise postpartum will depend on the type of delivery and postpartum state of the woman and should be left to the discretion of the woman's obstetrician. Once clearance is given to resume exercise, a time allowance of 180 days should be sufficient for the woman to meet physical fitness standards.

• The Healthy People 2000 (DHHS, 1991) goal for breastfeeding specifies that at least 75 percent of women should breastfeed their babies in the early postnatal period and 50 percent of women should continue to breastfeed until their babies are 5 to 6 months old. As the military has provided no indication as to why they should not strive to comply with this goal, the subcommittee recommends that efforts be made to promote and support breastfeeding among all servicewomen, where appropriate. Promotion of breastfeeding can be incorporated into prenatal classes, family support classes, hospital policies, and training of health care providers.

• The BCNH subcommittee calls attention to the persistent anemia and musculoskeletal and cardiovascular changes that may continue in some women postpartum. These changes may present potential health problems for the mother and compromise her fitness status. Women with low iron stores before pregnancy or excessive blood losses at delivery may require an extended period (5–10 months) to replete and normalize stores.

• An increase in the length of exemption from deployment from 4 to 6 months postpartum is recommended to support maternal postpartum recovery, breastfeeding, and enhanced infant health and development.

• The BCNH subcommittee acknowledges that childbearing is compatible with a military career when planning and education on effective birth control and counseling on the importance of timing pregnancy in one's military career are provided to all servicemembers. The subcommittee therefore recommends training and education for all supervisory personnel regarding pregnancy policy, as well as a prenatal counseling program for pregnant active-duty women. These policies should be implemented to reduce attrition and enhance military readiness.

RECOMMENDATIONS FOR FUTURE RESEARCH

Currently, there are no systematically collected data describing what military women do to meet weight and fitness standards (both before and after childbirth), how effective their behaviors are at maintaining weight and fitness standards, and the long-term health consequences of these behaviors. A DoD-wide evaluation system is recommended.

Survey Design and Administration

Relevant Data from Previous Surveys of Military Personnel and in Existing DoD Databases

Several research projects have been conducted by the services on the health-related behaviors of servicemembers. In addition to the wide variety of demographic and personnel data maintained in the Defense Manpower Data Center database, health outcome data are maintained in several medical cost accounting databases.

Effective Use of Existing Data

A combination of the survey instruments that have been used in the past would be suitable for collecting most of the information needed (including longitudinal data). The personnel and medical databases are capable of producing much of the remaining information needed. However, the subcommittee finds that there are two problems with this method of data collection. First, some of the survey data were collected anonymously (with no identification numbers of any type), precluding any attempt to examine the data longitudinally or merge the databases with existing personnel and medical databases that contain the demographic and health outcome data needed for a comprehensive analysis of the data. Second, the personnel and medical databases were not designed to be linked to each other or to survey databases. Thus, although much potentially worthwhile information is collected, little meaningful analysis can be performed.

Recommendations for New Methods

The subcommittee recommends that the military survey a representative sample of active-duty personnel individually and review the individuals' personnel and medical records during the course of the interview. This method would enable the investigator to obtain all the data needed in a single effort, ensure quality control of the data, build a database that would preserve the anonymity of the individual, and obviate the need to merge automated information systems with highly sensitive data. However, the need to create a system that will obtain information from several large and representative samples of the entire DoD over the course of several years may make this choice cost-prohibitive.

An alternative recommendation is to expand the triennial *Survey of Health-Related Behaviors among Military Personnel* to include the demographic, medical, nutrition, fitness, and pregnancy data needed. Changing the questionnaire to include social security number, as was done with the Navy's *Perceptions of Wellness and Readiness Assessment* survey and the Army's *Health Risk Appraisal* survey, would permit a longitudinal and potentially integrated database to be developed. The practice of using questions from federal surveys of health and fitness-related behaviors in the general U.S. population should be continued so that comparisons between military and civilian populations can be made.

Additional Data Needed

As recommended by an earlier IOM report (1992), longitudinal studies of people admitted to military weight management or remedial fitness programs should be conducted to determine the outcome of these programs as recommended changes in program procedures are implemented.

Career, active-duty, military women constitute a unique population of individuals who are required to maintain their weight and body fat and fitness at prescribed levels. Longitudinal studies of health risk factors (cardiovascular, musculoskeletal, metabolic) and outcomes are recommended for these women.

The DoD is encouraged to monitor pregnancy outcome (birthweight, preterm delivery, low birth weight and small-for-date infants, and congenital anomalies) as well as pregnancy wastage (miscarriage) according to service, rank, and MOS to identify potential problems associated with certain military jobs, physical training, or hazardous environments. Longitudinal studies are recommended on body weight and fitness of women who have given birth. It is recommended that health surveys be expanded to collect information on the pregnancy history of active-duty women. Suggested questions are those used by Evans and Rosen (1996).

Additional Research Recommendations

• Additional research is needed to refine and standardize anthropometric equations for body fat prediction and to validate them against current four-compartment models. This research must include a population that is representative of active-duty military women in ethnic and age profile.

• In view of the relationship between skeletal muscle/FFM and strength, and recent developments in the ability to assess these parameters, research is recommended to develop an expedient method for the prediction of FFM using anthropometric measurements.

• The use of standard military equations in postpartum women for estimating body fat at return-to-duty testing has not been validated. Therefore, the BCNH subcommittee recommends that validation studies be conducted in these women, controlling for ethnicity, age, and parity.

• Task assessment and redesign are recommended, where appropriate, to ensure gender-neutral accession and retention standards in individual MOSs.

, • Further research is recommended on the incidence and risk factors for stress fracture and other musculoskeletal injuries in active-duty women.

• Additional research is needed on the effects of environmental stressors on the nutritional status and needs of active-duty women. It is recommended that the military coordinate its research efforts in this area with those of the civilian sector.

REFERENCES

ACOG (American College of Obstetricians and Gynecologists). 1994. Exercise during pregnancy and the postpartum period. ACOG Technical Bulletin 189. February. Washington, D.C.: ACOG.

ACSM (American College of Sports Medicine). 1990. ACSM position stand. The recommended quantity and quality of exercise for developing and maintaining cardiorespiratory and muscular fitness in healthy adults. Med. Sci. Sports Exerc. 22:265–274.

AR (Army Regulation) 40-25. 1985. See U.S. Departments of the Army, the Navy, and the Air Force, 1985.

DHHS (U.S. Department of Health and Human Services). 1991. Healthy People 2000: National Health Promotion and Disease Prevention Objectives. DHHS (PHS) Publ. No. 91-50212. Public Health Service, U.S. Department of Health and Human Services. Washington, D.C.: U.S. Government Printing Office.

Evans, M.A., and L. Rosen. 1996. Women in the military: Pregnancy, command climate, organizational behavior, and outcomes. Technical Report No. HR 96-001, Part I, Defense Women's Health Research Program. Fort Sam Houston, Tx.: U.S. Army Medical Department Center and School.

IOM (Institute of Medicine). 1990. Nutrition during Pregnancy: Part I, Weight Gain; Part II, Nutrient Supplements. Subcommittee on Nutritional Status and Weight Gain during Pregnancy, Subcommittee on Dietary Intake and Nutrient Supplements during Pregnancy, Committee on Nutritional Status during Pregnancy and Lactation, Food and Nutrition Board. Washington, D.C.: National Academy Press.

IOM. 1991. Nutrition during Lactation. Subcommittee on Lactation, Committee on Nutritional Status during Pregnancy and Lactation, Food and Nutrition Board. Washington, D.C.: National Academy Press.

IOM 1992. Body Composition and Physical Performance, Applications for the Military Services, B.M. Marriott and J. Grumstrup-Scott, eds. Committee on Military Nutrition Research, Food and Nutrition Board. Washington, D.C.: National Academy Press.

IOM. 1998. Dietary Reference Intakes: Folate, Other B Vitamins, and Choline. Standing Committee on the Scientific Evaluation of Dietary Reference Intakes, Food and Nutrition Board. Washington, D.C.: National Academy Press.

Appendix J

Conclusions and Recommendations from the Brief Report Reducing Stress Fractures in Physically Active Military Women

Submitted June 1998

Subcommittee Responses to Questions, Conclusions, and Recommendations

As described in the Executive Summary of this report, the incidence of stress fractures during U.S. military basic training is significantly higher in female recruits than in male recruits. As part of the Defense Women's Health Program, the Subcommittee on Body Composition, Nutrition, and Health was requested to evaluate the effects of diet, genetics, and physical activity on bone mineral and calcium status in young servicewomen. The subcommittee provides the following conclusions and recommendations in response to the five questions posed by the military.

1. Why is the incidence of stress fractures in military basic training greater for women than for men?

Stress fracture rates among female Army military trainees during basic combat training are more than twice those reported for males (Deuster et al., 1997; Jones, 1996; MSMR, 1997). This greater incidence appears to be due in part to the initial entry level of fitness of the recruits and specifically the ability of bone to withstand the rapid, large increases in physical loading. The rate of increase in the intensity, frequency, or volume of impact of loading activities in basic training is a risk factor for stress fractures. In addition, increased stride length and variations in specific exercise activities may contribute to the different site distribution of stress fractures in military women compared with military men. When training regimens are equally imposed on men and women, the resultant stress on the less physically fit increases the likelihood of injury.

Conclusions

Low initial fitness of recruits appears to be the principal factor in the development of stress fractures during basic training. A key component of training programs should be to match closely the rate of musculoskeletal adaptation with the participant, in order to avoid interruption of training for cardiovascular and muscular endurance or fitness. In the training program for female soldiers, rapid and excessive increases in exercise habits and abrupt changes in training load may increase the risk of stress fractures of the lower extremities. The subcommittee concludes that muscle mass, strength, and resistance to fatigue with cyclic loading (bone stress created by excessive or rapid incremental skeletal muscle contraction and loading forces) play a critical role in development of stress fracture. To attain an adequate level of fitness, a training program must include a history of sufficient loading and remodeling within bone if stress injuries and fractures are to be prevented during periods of intense training. Proper footwear and appropriate choice of running surfaces also contribute to the prevention of injuries. Currently there may not be sufficient time during basic training to achieve the aerobic fitness level required to avoid musculoskeletal injury.

Recommendations

A more appropriate fitness standard should be achieved by women entering military service either through a structured program prior to their beginning basic training or through an integrated program within basic training. It is recommended that such a program be designed to start women at a lower level of activity and gradually increase their activity as a transition into full-scale basic training. If a prebasic training program is selected, it should utilize training techniques similar to those employed in basic training.

The BCNH subcommittee recommends a program of basic training that encourages and focuses on (1) avoiding training errors by alternating easy and hard days (i.e., substituting low or nonimpact loading for physical routines that lead to cardiopulmonary fitness), (2) gradual building of skeletal muscle mass with selected strength and endurance activities, and (3) identifying specific exercises that may modify the etiology and site distribution of stress fractures among women and provide ones that do not incur an increased risk for developing stress fractures.

2. What is the relationship of genetics and body composition to bone density and the incidence of stress fractures in women?

Genetics is a determinant of peak bone mass, but it is not known what genes are important nor is it known how important they are in the risk assessment profile for stress fractures.

Body mass and composition *per se* influence bone density. Greater body mass is associated with higher levels of bone mineral mass and density.

Stress fractures are associated not only with reduced skeletal muscle mass and its concomitant increased fatigability and lower fitness levels but also with an excessive skeletal muscle mass and its enhanced strength. Bone stress created by excessive or rapid incremental skeletal muscle contraction and loading forces can cause fractures at specific anatomic sites. However, the major problem for military recruits is likely to be insufficient muscle mass.

Conclusions

It is well recognized that the etiology of stress fracture is multifactorial and that lower bone mineral density is only one contributing factor. Genetics and body mass, specifically muscle mass, are also important determinants in the development of stress fractures. Although current technologies (e.g., dual energy x-ray absorptiometry [DXA], peripheral DXA [pDXA], quantitative computed tomography [QCT], peripheral QCT [pQCT], and ultrasound) may be useful for bone density assessment, which has a wide range of normal values, they cannot be used to screen for stress fracture.

Recommendations

Bone measurements should not be used routinely for screening recruits. Problems with the accuracy of bone mineral content measurements (both specificity and sensitivity) make it difficult to predict stress fractures in military women. Moreover, mean bone mineral density measurements among athletes with stress fracture lie within the normal range.

3. What are the effects of diet, physical activity, contraceptive use, and other lifestyle factors (smoking and alcohol) on the accrual of peak bone mineral content, incidence of stress fractures, and development of osteoporosis in military women?

Energy intake should be adequate (2,000–2,800 kcal/d) to maintain weight during moderate and intensive physical fitness training. A diet adequate in calcium, phosphorus, magnesium, and vitamin D (IOM, 1997) and moderate in sodium and protein (NRC, 1989) should optimize bone health in the short term and theoretically should reduce the long-term risk of developing osteoporosis.

Weight-bearing activity determines the shape and mass of bone. Graded increases in physical activity and resultant increases in the level of musculoskeletal fitness are necessary to ensure sufficient time for loading and remodeling within bone to prevent stress injuries and fractures.

The use of oral contraceptives that contain estrogen with or without progestogens is not considered to have long-term detrimental effects and may benefit bone health. Use of long-acting depot preparations of progestational agents, such as Depro-Provera, has been associated with relative estrogen deficiency. Long-term use of gonadotropin-releasing hormone agonists induces a state of estrogen deficiency and has been associated with bone loss. Cigarette smoking may be a long-term risk factor for the development of osteoporosis, whereas excessive alcohol consumption may be a risk factor in the short term for overall injuries. Whether these lifestyle factors are directly related to the development of stress fractures in the short term or are indirectly related through their long term influence on bone density is not known.

Conclusions

Energy intake by military women should be adequate to maintain weight during intense physical fitness training. Training regimens should provide for a gradual increase of load-bearing activities ("ramp-up"). Nutritional modification of diets of incoming recruits cannot effectively prevent stress fractures during the short term of basic training. The use of oral contraceptive agents is not contraindicated. Exogenous estrogen-progestogen hormones may positively affect peak bone mass reached in adulthood, which may be important for future fracture risks in contrast to the use of long-acting progestogens and gonadotropin-releasing hormone agonists.

Recommendations

Implement measures to ensure that energy intakes by military women are consistent and adequate to maintain weight during intense physical fitness training.

Shift emphasis of the program to one of continual physical fitness, which in turn will assist in the maintenance of weight, fat-free mass, and bone mass in all active servicemembers.

The BCNH subcommittee strongly suggests that the Department of Defense (DoD) consider joining with other federal agencies and programs to educate young adults about the importance of physical activity for health and well-being and to identify those individuals who might be at high risk for stress fracture.

This role should be consistent with the DoD's need to have a pool of recruits sufficiently fit for military training.

4. How do caloric restriction and disordered eating patterns affect hormonal balance and the accrual and maintenance of peak bone mineral content?

Caloric restriction or disordered eating may lead to a hormonal disruption that is associated with amenorrhea and an associated estrogen deficiency and loss of bone mineral content (IOM, 1998).

Conclusions

Conditions that induce estrogen deficiency from any cause (e.g., training regimen, diet, weight loss) may adversely affect the skeleton. It is likely that the maintenance of body weight is important in preventing the onset of secondary amenorrhea.

Recommendations

In active-duty servicemembers it is recommended that fitness and body composition assessments be performed frequently. At a minimum, body weight and composition should be evaluated more frequently than the current 6 month intervals. This would foster adherence to practices of healthy weight and physical fitness and decrease high risk, or disordered eating behaviors.

The prevalence and underlying causes of oligomenorrhea and amenorrhea should be assessed in women undergoing basic training and advanced training and on active duty. Young women in the military should be provided with information about the associations among the menstrual cycle, estrogen sufficiency (including use of contraceptives), bone health, and energy restriction.

5. How can the military best ensure that the dietary intakes of active-duty military women in training and throughout their military careers do not contribute to an increased incidence of stress fractures and osteoporosis?

Nutrition education programs are key to providing information and direction on the choice and nutrient content of appropriate foods. It is important that education programs for military women be aimed at their meeting requirements for total energy needs as well as for nutrients supportive of optimal bone health. With consumption of appropriately higher energy intakes matched to meet the demands of physical training and fitness, higher intakes of calcium should be promoted.

Women should strive to maintain a stable body weight within weight-range standards appropriate for their service and should refrain from episodes of repetitive dieting and weight loss so as not to disrupt normal hormonal rhythms (IOM, 1998). Weight within standard may be achieved through proper diet, selection of nutrient-dense foods, and participation in weight-bearing exercise activities. These measures will be beneficial for the reduction of stress fracture risk in the short term, as well as for osteoporosis prevention in the long term.

Conclusions

Many predisposing factors can alter the menstrual cycle. It is likely that maintenance of appropriate body weight is important in preventing the onset of secondary amenorrhea. To ensure adequate nutrient intakes, female military personnel must be educated on how to meet both energy and nutrient needs. This education is required to enable women to choose foods of higher nutrient density and to maintain a fitness program that will allow greater energy intake.

Recommendations

As recommended in its previous report (IOM, 1998), the BCNH subcommittee "reinforces the requirement for adequate energy and nutrient intakes to reflect the needs of the body at a moderate activity level (2,000–2,800 kcal/d) . . . The subcommittee reinforces the recent efforts of the Army to begin providing complete nutritional labeling of all ration components and to include information to enable identification of nutrient-dense components that would help women meet the MRDAs (Military Recommended Dietary Allowances) at their usual energy intake. . . . The subcommittee recommends nutritional labeling of all dining hall menu items and provision of food selection guidelines to women in garrison" (p. 162).

The military should develop aggressive education programs for military women aimed at helping them identify and select appropriate foods and fortified food products to increase the number of women meeting their requirements for these nutrients. If nutrition education and counseling sessions fail to promote increased intakes, the use of calcium-fortified products becomes essential. Calcium supplements should be recommended under appropriate guidance by the military to meet women's special needs.

RECOMMENDATIONS FOR
FUTURE RESEARCH BY THE MILITARY

• Research is needed to define the appropriate fitness level that is required to enable a woman to enter and participate in basic training without incurring an increased risk of stress fractures.

• Data on initial fitness levels should be compiled in recruits from all military services by age, gender, and race/ethnicity.

• Further study is needed to determine the types of activities that may predispose women to stress fractures, especially in the pelvic region and upper leg, and steps should be taken to modify their activities in basic training to lower risk.

• Stress fracture incidence statistics should be collected by age, gender, race/ethnicity, and skeletal site, using a gender-independent, standardized definition of stress fracture and a comparable time frame from all military services for both the basic training and posttraining periods.

• Military research efforts should contribute to identifying those factors, such as diet, lifestyle, and ethnicity, that may contribute to achieving peak bone mass, as well as components of military programs that may interfere with this process.

• Efforts should be made, particularly in women, to investigate more fully the now-preliminary linkages between low skeletal muscle mass and stress fracture risk. Investigators should attempt to determine if this relationship is due to a low skeletal muscle mass effect *per se* or an associated factor such as inadequate initial fitness status.

• Research is needed on the effects of implanted or injectable contraceptives, such as Depo-Provera, on bone mineral density and bone strength. Chemical formulation, dosage, and route of administration require further investigation.

• Research is needed that assesses the effect of dietary energy status of military women on the secretion of hormones that affect bone health, particularly in situations of high metabolic stress.

• The military should continue to gather dietary intake data and evidence concerning calcium intakes throughout the soldier's career, as training programs, food choices, and food supply change over time.

• Based on preliminary data from athletes, the potential loss of calcium in sweat due to physical exertion during training and the impact of high levels of activity on calcium requirements needs to be investigated as possible pathophysiological factors in the development of stress fracture.

• More research is needed to evaluate existing technologies for cost-effective assessment of bone mass. These technologies currently include ultrasound, central and peripheral dual-energy x-ray absorptiometry, and central and peripheral quantitative computer tomography. Ultimately, the cost-benefit analysis of all techniques will have to be addressed for specific uses and populations within the military.

• Mechanical models should be developed which link skeletal muscle mass, force/torque, and bone stress in humans, as well as to improve existing in vivo methods of quantifying components of these models.

REFERENCES

Deuster, P.A., B.H. Jones, and J. Moore. 1997. Patterns and risk factors for exercise-related injuries in women: a military perspective. Mil. Med. 162:649–655.

IOM (Institute of Medicine). 1997. Dietary Reference Intakes for Calcium, Phosphorus, Magnesium, Vitamin D, and Fluoride [prepublication copy]. Standing Committee on the Scientific Evaluation of Dietary Reference Intakes, Food and Nutrition Board. Washington, D.C.: National Academy Press.

IOM. 1998. Assessing Readiness in Military Women: The Relationship to Body Composition, Nutrition, and Health. Committee on Body Composition, Nutrition, and Health of Military Women, Committee on Military Nutrition Research, Food and Nutrition Board. Washington, D.C.: National Academy Press.

Jones, B.H. 1996. Injuries among women and men in gender integrated BCT units Fort Leonard Wood 1995. Med. Surveill. Mon. Rep. 2(2):2–3, 7–8.

MSMR (Medical Surveillance Monthly Report). 1997. Spontaneous fractures of the femur, active-duty soldiers. 3:2–9.

NRC (National Research Council). 1989. Diet and Health: Implications for Reducing Chronic Disease Risk. Committee on Diet and Health, Food and Nutrition Board, Commission on Life Sciences. Washington, D.C.: National Academy Press.

Appendix K

Letter Report:
Antioxidants and Oxidative Stress in Military Personnel

Submitted February 12, 1999

INSTITUTE OF MEDICINE
NATIONAL ACADEMY OF SCIENCES
2101 CONSTITUTION AVENUE, N.W.   WASHINGTON, DC 20418

February 12, 1999

Maj. General John Parker
Commander
U.S. Army Medical Research
  and Materiel Command
504 Scott Street
Fort Detrick, MD 21702-5012

Dear General Parker:

At the request of MAJ Vicky Thomas, MS, RD, Nutrition Staff Officer, Office of the Surgeon General, and LTC Karl Friedl, Ph.D., Program Director, Army Operational Medicine, U.S. Army Medical Research and Materiel Command (USAMRMC) and Grant Officer Representative of USAMRMC for Grant No. DAMD17-94-J-4046 to the National Academy of Sciences for support of the Food and Nutrition Board's (FNB) Committee on Military Nutrition Research (CMNR), members of CMNR met in Washington, D.C. on July 29-31, 1998.

The Office of the Surgeon General (OSG), through USAMRMC, requested that CMNR provide interim guidance on the potential value of supplemental antioxidants for the health and readiness of service members. The questions posed by the OSG related to the value of specific supplements (Vitamins C, E and β-carotene) administered proactively to protect individuals against hazards in the military environment which may not be typical of exposures in the general U.S. population. This issue was to be addressed with a one day workshop (including presentations from outside experts, as appropriate) and a rapid turnaround letter report conveying the committee's conclusions and recommendations.

Further, the USAMRMC was aware of the ongoing activity of a FNB panel currently working to develop Dietary Reference Intakes (DRIs) for dietary antioxidants and related compounds which has the broader objective of defining nutrient intakes to promote health and decrease risk of chronic disease in the general population. Thus, in the Task Statement, USAMRMC limited its request to concerns for individuals in the military environment, which may not be typical of exposures in the general population. The CMNR was not to address whether supplements of vitamins E, C, and ß-carotene may protect service members against chronic disease but was to consider the short-term antioxidant effects that may be only tenuously linked to chronic disease.

231

The CMNR was particularly pleased to have Lt. Gen. Ronald Blanck, Surgeon General of the U.S. Army attend the workshop, and provide further elaboration of his interest and that of the Medical Command in promoting the health of military personnel and their dependents beyond the traditional role of providing medical treatment services.

The primary concern of the OSG, and thus the focus of the Task Statement, is the evaluation of potential oxidative stress exposures of military personnel which are believed to be high as a consequence of some occupational-specific demands (e.g., high intensity work) and working environments (e.g., exposures to air pollutants during deployments to some parts of the world). The consequences of such exposures may include acute effects on suppression of immune function indices and possibly increased susceptibility to infectious disease and/or reduced capacity to respond to immunizations, as discussed in the CMNR report *Military Strategies for Sustainment of Nutrition and Immune Function in the Field* (IOM, 1999). Physical capacity may be diminished through oxidative stress effects, at least in the specific case of work at altitude (*Nutritional Needs in Cold and High-Altitude Environments,* IOM, 1996). Long-term health consequences, including progression of neurodegenerative diseases, may result from low level toxins, radio frequencies, and psychological stress exposures; these have been postulated to operate through oxidative stress mechanisms. Given the many suspected links between oxidative stress and health and performance, the CMNR was asked to determine if it would be prudent to provide supplements of β-carotene, vitamin C, and vitamin E to service members rather than wait for conclusive research results. The decision to supplement would depend, in part, on what risks are known to be associated with high intakes of these substances, and on the strength of the evidence that these may be of any benefit to service members, whether through antioxidant properties or through other effects. Specifically, the CMNR was requested to address the following three key questions:

1. What is the strength of the evidence to suggest that oxidative stress is a concern for service members during extremes of physical activity and other stresses encountered in training and operations?

2. What is the strength of the evidence that vitamin C, vitamin E, and/or β-carotene are likely to protect health and performance of service members exposed to multiple environmental stresses during military training and operations (e.g. severe air pollution in some urban environments; radiation hazards to crew at altitude; radio frequency radiation hazards on ships and around communications facilities; lung and tissue blast overpressure effects and physical and psychological stresses in extreme training courses such as Ranger training and USMC crucible training)?

3. Is there evidence of any health risk associated with supplementing intakes of vitamin C, vitamin E, and β-carotene by service members, with the intention of maintaining health and performance in adverse military training and operational environments?

A workshop developed to assist the CMNR in a review of the state of scientific knowledge to address these issues was held immediately following another FNB sponsored workshop that examined issues related to the selection of appropriate biomarkers for assessing nutritional status of the general population in relation to dietary antioxidant and related compounds, and critical adverse effects that might be used to determine tolerable upper intake levels of vitamins E, C, the carotenoids and selenium. Thus the CMNR was able to obtain much additional information on the antioxidant compounds of specific interest to the Surgeon General.

This report has two parts. Part I is this letter that contains the conclusions and general recommendations of the CMNR. Part II includes two attachments. Attachment A is the answers to the specific questions posed by the Army representatives with pertinent references. Attachment B contains the workshop agenda, list of speakers, and abstracts of the presentations.

This report of the CMNR has been reviewed in accordance with National Research Council guidelines by a separate scientific review panel whose membership is listed in Attachment A. The report is based on executive session discussions by the Committee and is a thoughtfully developed presentation incorporating the scientific opinion of the CMNR and the comments of the peer review panel.

CONCLUSIONS AND RECOMMENDATIONS

The CMNR commends the Surgeon General for promoting efforts to move military medicine into a preventive mode rather than focusing almost entirely on treatment concerns. There are aspects of military service that may enhance overall health compared with that of the general public. The two most notable aspects are required exercise relating to maintaining physical fitness, and maintenance of desirable weight as specified by the weight [body composition] standards.

It is also quite clear that proactive lifestyle changes have by far the greatest potential for improving the overall health of military personnel and their dependents beyond any benefits that might be identified from supplemental antioxidant use. Estimates of the major health benefits that accompany lifestyle changes include: (1) cessation of smoking: a 50-70% reduced risk of heart disease; (2) the reduction of blood cholesterol from 220 to 198: a 20-30 % reduced risk of heart disease; and (3) pharmocologic therapy for diastolic blood pressures over 90 mm Hg - a 16% reduction in risk of heart disease and a 42 % lower risk of stroke. Moderation of alcohol intake, adequate exercise, maintenance of a desirable weight, and consuming diets consistent with the Dietary Guidelines for Americans (USDA, 1995) have all been shown to provide substantial benefits greater than any potential value of supplemental antioxidants. (Hennekens, 1998; DHHS, 1991).

The CMNR presents the following conclusions and recommendations to the Surgeon General, and the U.S. Army Medical Research and Materiel Command regarding the benefits and risks of supplementing military personnel with vitamins C, E and β-carotene for protection from militarily unique situations of oxidative stress.

Conclusions

Information presented at this meeting, in earlier CMNR reports, and other scientific literature provide evidence that military service leads to exposure to unique oxidative stresses that may have adverse health consequences. Some of these stresses are reasonably well characterized, such as those associated with strenuous exercise, work in extremes of environmental temperatures, and at altitude. Much less is known about other sources of oxidative stress, such as radiofrequency and microwave radiation hazards, exposure to blast overpressure, and psychological stress related to extreme training courses or deployment.

The multiple occupational stresses associated with military tasks often occur together in deployment situations. These stresses may have more severe effects as food intake becomes more limited; thus, those individuals with both diminished food intake and high stress would be the most likely target population. Among them, those exposed to these adverse conditions for extended periods of time might be the most vulnerable.

Military personnel living on military bases and those in deployment situations have access to diets that are formulated according to the Military Recommended Dietary Allowances (MRDA). The MRDAs provide guidance for recommended daily intakes of nutrients, based on the National Research Council's Recommended Dietary Allowances (NRC, 1980). Studies of military personnel living in garrison reveal satisfactory dietary intakes of vitamin C (averaging 2x the MRDA). Vitamin E intakes measured in four studies indicated that in three of the locations evaluated, median intakes were equal to or greater than the MRDA of 10 mg. However, one study of Army Rangers at Fort Stewart indicated a median vitamin E intake of only 6.9 mg/ day (Corey Baker Fulco, U.S. Army Research Institute of Environmental Medicine, personal communication, July 17, 1998).

Military rations formulated in accordance with the MRDAs provide nutrients in amounts consistent with meeting nutrient needs—including the antioxidant nutrients—when these rations are consumed at levels required to maintain body weight in the usual range of physical activity for military task requirements. There is little evidence that supplementation with vitamins C, E or with β-carotene in normal conditions (i.e. in garrison) would enhance overall health.

In contrast to garrison situations, the CMNR recognizes that there are circumstances where the various environmental and emotional stresses of military operations may result in a tendency to reduce ration intake. Studies carried out in field training exercises consistently demonstrate that caloric intake is reduced to approximately 75% of troops' usual intakes. In basic training, negative energy balance and weight loss also occur, probably as a result of both decreased energy intake and greatly increased energy expenditure. Such situations may be associated with intakes of vitamins C, E, and β-carotene (vitamin A) below recommended levels. In the report, *Not Eating Enough* (IOM, 1995), the CMNR proposed establishing a Food Doctrine with suggestions of how to minimize the underconsumption of rations in the field in order to reduce the impact of these environmental factors on food intake and consequent overall nutrient intake. The committee recognizes there may be some benefit to enhancing body reserves of these nutrients prior to deployment but at current levels of reported consumption, body stores have not been evaluated.

There is little evidence currently available to indicate that supplementation of vitamins C and E and β-carotene would be beneficial in protecting against short term, acute oxidative stress. In addition, the use of antioxidant compounds to minimize this stress is not without risk.

Trials reviewed by the committee in which supplemental β-carotene was given to smokers appeared to increase the risk of lung cancer. These data are especially relevant since a large segment of the military population still engages in smoking. Recent studies from the National Institutes of Health (NIH) indicate that daily intakes of 100 mg of vitamin C saturated circulating immune cells and was reflective of other body tissues. Furthermore, as intake exceeded 100 mg per day, bioavailability decreased and above 500 mg, the entire absorbed dose was excreted. Thus there appears to be little benefit in intakes of vitamin C above 100 mg. In fact, the value of intake levels adequate to provide saturation of tissues has not been clarified. There is also some evidence that high levels of vitamin E (400 to 800 mg/day) inhibit platelet aggregation, and when taken with non-steroidal anti-inflammatory medication can result in excessive bleeding which would be a particular concern for injured or wounded personnel. Data which the committee considered important in making recommendations are detailed in Part II, Attachment A of this report.

RECOMMENDATIONS

Based on the review and discussion of information presented at the July 29-31, 1998 meeting, recent scientific literature, and previous reports prepared by CMNR , the committee recommends that:

• Effective methods of promoting lifestyle changes as outlined in *Diet and Health* (NRC, 1989), *Healthy People 2000* (DHHS, 1991) and *Healthy People*

2010 (in draft) be developed as these have the greatest potential of maintaining health and performance of military personnel and their dependents, particularly in view of the introductory comments of Lt. General Blanck concerning the transition of military medicine to a health promotion emphasis.

• Aggressive educational efforts be directed to military personnel engaged in operations of various intensities and in stressful environments on the importance of striving to maintain food intakes consistent with physical demands and energy requirements to avoid excessive weight loss.

• Emphasis be placed on meeting the recommendations of the Dietary Guidelines for Americans (USDA/DHHS, 1995) rather than supplementing with individual nutrients.

• Supplementation should not be considered except in specific high stress situations where intake is likely to be markedly inadequate. If supplementation is determined to be necessary, however, data on the benefits of doses exceeding 100 mg/day of vitamin C and 50 mg/day of vitamin E as alpha tocopherol are not definitive and need to be confirmed. Supplementation of β-carotene for military personnel is **NOT** recommended at this time.

• As study results become available in trials of the interrelationships of vitamin E and vitamin C to muscle soreness and to immunological function, these recommendations should be reviewed again.

Future Research Considerations

The CMNR believes that the military services, through their pool of volunteer personnel, have an excellent and often unique opportunity to generate statistics about nutrition, health, and well-being of service personnel that can be directly applied toward improved health of both military personnel and the general U.S. population. Research on the following topics is recommended.

• Research focused on the protective effects of antioxidants against acute oxidative stress is strongly encouraged as information is most lacking in this area.

• Validation of a battery of biomarkers for detecting oxidative tissue damage in human subjects in ambulatory or field situations.

• Evaluation of the extent to which the presence of tissue oxidative damage impacts performance.

• The extent and duration of oxidative stress that might be associated with hyperoxia, prolonged exposure to ionizing radiation, radiofrequency, blast overpressure, and psychological stress.

• Supplementation of vitamins C, E and β-carotene in a controlled, randomized way so that their true efficacy in decreasing oxidative tissue damage based on validated biomarkers can be determined. This research is essential both with respect to optimizing health and performance of personnel, and optimizing cost effectiveness.

The CMNR is pleased to provide this review as part of the Committee's continuing response to the U.S. Army Medical Research and Materiel Command. The Committee always welcomes comments and suggestions from you or your staff regarding how these reports can better serve the Army.

Sincerely,

John E. Vanderveen, Ph.D. (Chair)
Lawrence E. Armstrong, Ph.D.
William R. Beisel, M.D
Gail E. Butterfield, Ph.D., R.D.
Wanda Chenoweth, Ph.D., R.D.
Johanna T. Dwyer, D.Sc., R.D.
John D. Fernstrom, Ph.D.
Robin B. Kanarek, Ph.D.
Orville A. Levander, Ph.D.
Esther M. Sternberg, M.D.
Douglas W. Wilmore, M.D.

Attachments
cc: LTG Ronald Blanck
       LTC Karl Friedl
       MAJ Vicky Thomas
       Kenneth Shine
       Susanne Stoiber
       Allison Yates
       Mary Poos

REFERENCES

DHHS (Department of Health and Human Services). 1991. Healthy People 2000: National Health Promotion and Disease Prevention Objectives. DHHS Publication No. (PHS) 91-50213. Washington, D.C.: U.S. Government Printing Office.

Hennekens, C.H. 1998. Antioxidant Vitamins: Current and Future Directions. Presented at IOM Workshop: *Antioxidants and the Effects of Oxidative Stress in Military Personnel.* July 30, 1998. Washington, D.C.

IOM (Institute of Medicine). 1993. Nutritional Needs in Hot Environments. B. Marriott (ed.). Washington, D.C.: National Academy Press.

IOM. 1995. Not Eating Enough. B. Marriott (ed.). Washington D.C.: National Academy Press

IOM. 1996. Nutritional Needs in Cold and High Altitude Environments. B. Marriott and S.J. Carlson (eds.). Washington, D.C. National Academy Press.

IOM. 1999. Military Strategies for Sustainment of Nutrition and Immune Function in the Field. Washington, D.C: National Academy Press (in press)

NRC (National Research Council. 1980. Recommended Dietary Allowances, 9th Edition. Washington D.C.: National Academy Press

NRC (National Research Council). 1989. Diet and Health: Implications for Reducing Chronic Disease Risk. Washington, D.C.: National Academy Press.

USDA (U.S. Department of Agriculture) and DHHS. 1995. Nutrition and Your Health: Dietary Guidelines for Americans, Fourth Edition. Home and Garden Bulletin No. 232. Washington, D.C.: U.S. Government Printing Office.

A

Answers to the Three Specific Questions Presented to the CMNR by Army Representatives

The responses to the three specific questions posed to the CMNR are:

1. What is the strength of the evidence to suggest that oxidative stress is a concern for service members during extremes of physical activity and other stresses encountered in military training or in the field?

Oxidative stress is a pathophysiological process in which the balance between pro-oxidants and antioxidants is shifted toward pro-oxidants. Strenuous physical exercise is associated with increased production of reactive oxygen species (pro-oxidants) in various tissues as well as a decline in levels of antioxidants (Sen, 1995; Kanter, 1998). The impact of this shift on health and physical performance is not well defined. However, the relatively consistent finding of an increase in antioxidant enzyme activity in the tissues of trained subjects (Alessio and Goldfarb, 1988; Hameren et al, 1993) suggests a protective adaptation to the habitual stress of exercise. Furthermore, it has been demonstrated that one of the most sensitive markers for exercise-induced oxidative stress, blood glutathione oxidation, returns to normal levels within 24 hr post-exercise in adequately nourished individuals (Sen et al, 1994).

Exercise is a daily part of military life. Depending on the intensity of the exercise, oxidative stress may become a factor. Routine conditioning provides general health benefits that may include some enhancement of ability to deal with subsequent oxidative stress. Although military assignments generally do not involve this type of stress, some duty assignments do involve extremes of exercise which can increase oxidative stress. Examples of military scenarios which would likely result in oxidative stresses severe enough to overwhelm the antioxidant defense mechanisms include battle operations, Ranger/Seals training, basic inductee training, and mobilization of reservists into active duty assignments.

239

To determine the strength of the scientific evidence that oxidative stress is a concern for military personnel during extremes of physical activity, the following issues must be considered: (1) Evidence that prolonged or high-intensity exercise bouts increase muscle-tissue free radicals, muscle tissue nitric oxide (NO, a powerful oxidant), conversion of xanthine dehydrogenase to xanthine oxidase, and conversion of glutathione (GSH) to glutathione disulfide (GS-SG); (2) Evidence that these forms of exercise simultaneously decrease tissue/blood levels of antioxidants, resulting in increased oxidation products and decreased protective biological antioxidants that could potentially lead to a situation of unopposed oxidative damage; (3) Evidence in laboratory animals and *in vitro* cell culture systems that such pro-oxidants cause lipid peroxidation, protein oxidation, and leukocyte DNA damage; (4) The availability and validity of biomarkers for detecting oxidative tissue damage in human subjects in ambulatory or field situations is not clear. No consensus exists regarding the overall value or accuracy of any of the markers currently used as indicators of total body or individual tissue levels of oxidative stress or damage. Biomarkers in breath, blood, urine, and biopsy specimens have been studied. Biomarkers in breath are easy to collect, especially in field conditions; these include measurements of pentane and aldehydes. Pentane analyses may have some value although standardization under various conditions needs to be improved. Biomarkers in blood include plasma lipid peroxides, glutathione, and xanthine oxidase. Urine biomarkers include malondialdehyde, 4-hydroxynonenal, 8-hydroxydeoxyguanosine and F_2-isoprostanes (Seis, 1986; Janero, 1990; Collins et al., 1996; Patrono and Fitzgerald, 1997). Different markers and timing of samples provide different results. For this reason, a battery of markers might be valuable if such markers can be validated.

There is evidence that in addition to strenuous physical activity during basic combat training, special forces training, or field operations, military personnel may also be exposed to other oxidative stresses when carrying out these physical activities in both hot and cold environmental temperature extremes, and at altitude. These additional oxidative stresses include hypoxia and extensive exposure to high intensity UV radiation from sunlight, and light reflection from snow or sand (Askew, 1995; Clarkson, 1993; Simon-Schnass, 1996). Strenuous activity under these conditions is frequently accompanied by reduced food intake, thus further reducing the availability of antioxidant nutrients (IOM, 1995).

A number of studies have been conducted to determine the effects of vitamin E supplementation on endurance exercise performance. In two studies of trained swimmers, swimming speed was not affected by vitamin E supplementation (Lawrence et al., 1975; Sharman et al., 1976). Physical performance of racing cyclists was also not improved by supplementation of 330 mg/day vitamin E for five months although serum creatine kinase and serum levels of malondialdehyde were significantly reduced in the vitamin E supplemented group (Rokitzki et al., 1994). Effects of vitamin E on tissue damage and physical performance has been studied in mountain climbers.

Prolonged exposure to physical exertion at high altitudes resulted in significantly increased breath pentane output and decreased physical performance as measured by a decrease in anaerobic threshold in unsupplemented climbers compared to climbers supplemented with 400 mg/day of vitamin E (Simon-Schnass and Pabst, 1988)

Another study, involving eight adult males, investigated the effect of vitamin E supplementation on DNA damage of peripheral white blood cells following a single bout of exhaustive exercise. Short term vitamin E supplementation (800 mg given at 12 and 2 hours pre- and 22 hr post-exercise) reduced DNA strand breakage associated with strenuous exercise. When subjects were supplemented with 1200 mg vitamin E/day for 14 days prior to exercise, DNA damage was significantly reduced (Hartman et al., 1995)

Several studies indicated some benefit of supplemental vitamin C in acclimation to work in hot environments, but Clarkson (1993) has questioned whether similar results would be found in better-nourished populations than the South African mine workers who were the subjects of those studies. Reynolds (1996), in an interpretive review of the effects of cold and altitude on vitamin and mineral requirements, concluded that there is a lack of research in these situations to establish a need for these nutrients above current recommended dietary allowances.

Musculoskeletal injuries have a greater impact on health and readiness of the U.S. Army than any other medical complaint during peacetime or combat. Reynolds et al. (1994) reported that these types of injuries (i.e., sprains, strains, and musculoskeletal pain) resulted in limited duty periods on average of 16.7 days, 3.0 days and 2.8 days per injury respectively. However, very little research has been done to determine if performance decrements are associated with the observed increases in markers of oxidative damage following strenuous exercise. Jakeman and Maxwell (1993) measured muscle contractile function using maximum voluntary contractions (MVC) and tetanic stimulation before and after eccentric exercise, and for 7 days during recovery. Their data suggested that prior supplementation with vitamin C, but not vitamin E (400mg/d for 21 days prior to exercise), may exert a protective effect against muscle damage induced by eccentric exercise. Francis and Hoobler (1986) also found no benefit of vitamin E in improving muscle soreness, range of motion, or peak muscle torque following exhaustive eccentric exercise. Using biomarkers of oxidative stress, Meydani et al. (1993) found a protective effect of vitamin E (800 mg/day for 48 days prior to exercise) on exercise-induced oxidative damage in both young and older adults, but did not examine any functional measures of muscle damage or performance indicators.

Additional research is needed to determine supplementation effects on performance decrements, timing of supplementation prior to exposure, level of supplementation, and duration of supplementation.

2. What is the strength of the evidence that Vitamin C, Vitamin E and/or β-carotene are likely to protect health and performance of service members exposed to multiple environmental stresses during military operations (e.g. severe air pollution in some urban environments; radiation hazards to air crews at altitude; radiofrequency radiation hazards on ships and around communications facilities; lung and tissue effects of blast overpressure; and physical and psychological stresses in extreme training courses such as Ranger training and USMC crucible training)?

The occupational hazards that military personnel encounter are heterogeneous. Many situations experienced by military personnel may increase oxidative stress. In addition to exercise, military duty includes various forms of stress likely to increase risk of oxidative exposure and potential injury in the following categories:

• Physical exposures: hypoxia, vibration, blast overpressure, lasers, G-forces, hyperoxia, weightlessness, microwaves, UV radiation, nuclear radiation, and continuous physical duty;
• Chemical exposures: cigarette smoking, toxic chemicals, and air/water pollution;
• Physiological conditions: undernutrition, sleep deprivation, immune activation associated with trauma, perfusion/reperfusion injury, wound healing, inflammation, and infectious illness; and
• Psychological: separation from family members, novel environments, fear/anxiety-provoking situations (e.g., dangerous mission assignments), role conflicts, threat of attack, and constant performance evaluation.

Some of these risks can be reduced or prevented by occupational health measures (protection from UV light exposure, from blast overpressure etc.). Others are innately related to military tasks. Moreover, the multiple occupational stresses associated with military tasks often occur together in conflict-related duty, and these stresses may have more severe effects as food becomes more limited. Thus, those individuals with both diminished food intake and high stress are the most likely target population for supplementation. Among them, those who are exposed to these adverse conditions for extended periods of time might be most vulnerable, although the scientific evidence is not as well defined for these other types of stress as for extreme exercise.

Figure 1 presents a theoretical scale describing the various situations which could occur among military personnel with respect to adequacy of food intake and exposure to environmental stresses which may lead to or be associated with acute oxidative stress. The shaded area under the curve represents where the combination of stressors and reduced intake could lead to inadequate antioxidant intake. Military personnel exposed to multiple stresses in situations of restricted food intake (e.g. special operations in a combat theater) would be at greatest

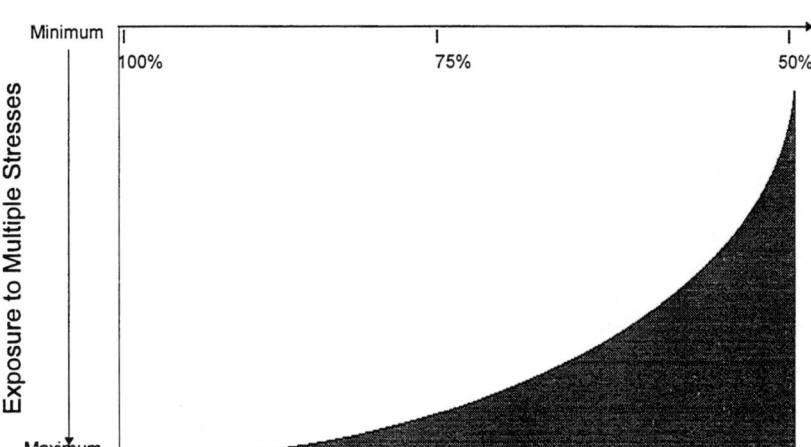

FIGURE 1 Conceptual relationship between food intake, stress exposure, and the potential need for supplemental antioxidants. Individuals with the lowest intakes and greatest stress exposure would be most likely to benefit from supplementation as indicated by the shaded area under the curve.

risk, and thus could potentially benefit from supplementation, while those meeting their caloric requirements in situations of minimum stress (e. g. routine duties in garrison) would be at minimal risk.

Under normal circumstances in garrison the members of the armed services have access to and consume a diet based on the Military Recommended Dietary Allowances (MRDA). Studies of military personnel living on and off base reveal generally satisfactory dietary intakes of vitamins C, but a summary of data from six intake surveys at different military installations indicated that in all but one survey, median vitamin A/β-carotene intakes were below the MRDA. Median vitamin E intakes were equal to or slightly above the MRDA of 10 mg in 3 of 4 studies, but the 4th study which involved Rangers indicated median vitamin E intakes of only 6.9 mg per day (Corey Baker-Fulco, USARIEM, July 17, 1998, personal communication). Little evidence exists that supplementation in non-stress conditions would enhance overall health, however.

In contrast to garrison situations, studies carried out during field training exercises consistently demonstrate that caloric intake is reduced to approximately 75% or less of troops' usual intakes (IOM, 1993; 1995). Several published military studies have documented immune dysregulation and suppression coupled with increased infections in soldiers participating in the Special Forces Assessment Schools (SFAS) and Ranger Training (Moore et al., 1992; Shippee et al., 1994; Bernton et al., 1995). Negative energy balance and weight loss occurs in these training situations, as well as in basic combat training, probably as a result of both decreased energy intake and greatly increased energy expenditure. Such situations may be associated with intakes of vitamin C, E, and β-carotene (as precursor of vitamin A) below recommended levels. Information about serum or tissue vitamin levels under these training and/or combat conditions is more limited.

In a two week study of Special Forces personnel, a treatment drink providing approximately 15 mg β-carotene, 400 mg α-tocopherol, 500 mg ascorbic acid and 100 mcg of selenium per day was compared to a placebo control. Serum levels of E and C were maintained, whereas on the placebo, serum vitamin E levels were maintained but ascorbic acid levels declined; β-carotene changes were not reported. In that study, antioxidant supplementation minimized immune dysfunction as measured by lymphocyte proliferation, but had little effect on delayed skin test hypersensitivity.

Preliminary unpublished data from a second study by the same investigators using a novel nutritional supplement containing these vitamins, as well as zinc, copper, structured lipid (triglycerides synthesized from a mixture of medium- and long-chain fatty acids) and other nutrients indicated more positive immune effects, including reduced anergy, increased proliferation after mitogen stimulation, and reduced incidence of upper respiratory infections in those receiving the supplement (Wood et al. Ross Laboratories, personal communication, July 30, 1998). Unfortunately, use of such a complex supplement precludes attributing benefit to the individual antioxidant compounds, but underscores the fact that it may be the interactions among nutrients that provide beneficial effects.

High altitude and cold stress (which increases energy output) have been studied in limited circumstances. The CMNR has recently reviewed these studies in depth (IOM, 1996). Although questions have been raised about increased needs for vitamin C and other nutrients in cold and high altitude environments, with the possible exception of vitamin E, there is little scientific basis at this time to indicate that cold or altitude exposures change the nutritional requirements for any vitamins or minerals. The MRDAs supply liberal amounts of these nutrients and should meet these needs. Although preliminary studies of increasing vitamin E intakes to 400 mg α-tocopherol per day showed promise in providing protective effects at high altitude, additional research is needed before questions regarding efficacy and effective doses are fully addressed and before implementing a supplement policy. Preliminary results of studies conducted at the Marine Mountain Warfare Training Center indicate a positive effect of a mixture of antioxidants (C, E, β-carotene, zinc, and selenium) in reducing oxidative stress as measured by breath pentane, whereas vitamins C, E, and β-carotene administered individually had no effect (E. Wayne Askew, Utah State University, personal communication, July 30, 1998).

Another source of stress relatively unique to military personnel is that of blast overpressure. Blast overpressure is the abrupt, rapid rise in atmospheric pressure resulting from explosive detonation, firing of large caliber weapons or accidental occupational explosions. This shock wave of air causes physical damage, mostly to the hollow organs such as ear, lung, and intestinal tract, but can also damage solid organs. The amount of damage is proportional to the peak pressure generated by the blast. The biochemical tissue damage has been shown to be a result of free radical reactions leading to oxidative stress as evidenced by increases in plasma lipid peroxidation products (thiobarbituric acid reactive substances (TBARS) and conjugated dienes), coupled with declines in blood levels of vitamins C, E, and glutathione (Elsayed et al., 1997, Elsayed, 1997). Significant changes were noted one hour following exposure, with tissue damage continuing to increase up to 24 hr after exposure. *In vitro* studies of lung and blood tissue removed from animals exposed to blast overpressure demonstrated that tissue levels of tocopherol declined rapidly and immediately, while tissue levels of glutathione and ascorbic acid did not show significant decline until 60 minutes post-exposure. However, addition of ascorbic acid or glutathione to the tissue medium actually increased tissue damage. Thus there is evidence that providing supplemental antioxidants after exposure may be detrimental. Preliminary data were presented to the committee from a follow-up study by these same investigators that provided pharmacological doses of either vitamin E (800 mg as α-tocopherol), vitamin C (1000 mg) or lipoic acid (25 mg) daily to rats for three days preceding blast exposure. The preliminary data showed a protective effect of vitamin E supplementation at this level prior to exposure, but vitamin C was not protective (Nabil Elsayed, Walter Reed Army Institute for Research, personal communication, July 30, 1998).

Microwave and radiofrequency wave exposure is another potential source of oxidative stress for military personnel. Military uses of microwaves include communications, radar and ultra-wide band (UWB) detection, signal jamming, electronic disabling, physical disruption (high power microwave systems) and Extremely Low Frequency (ELF) which includes electrical power main frequencies of 50-60 hertz. In humans, maximum absorption of microwaves occurs between 50 and 150 megahertz, which is the radiofrequency range. There is evidence from a wide variety of studies that link exposure to radiofrequency (electromagnetic fields) to increases in oxidative stress indicated by increased levels of nitric oxide and peroxynitrite, altered calcium metabolism, decreases in melatonin levels, and increased DNA strand breaks in (rat) brain tissue. Several recent epidemiological studies have indicated a link between occupational exposure to electromagnetic fields and increased risk of neurodegenerative disease, both Alzheimer's and ALS (Sobel et al., 1995; 1996; Gunnarsson et al., 1992; Davanipour et al., 1997). A recent study with Air Force personnel demonstrated an increase in risk of brain tumors from occupational exposure to electromagnetic radiation (Grayson, 1996). There is no information available concerning the potential of supplemental antioxidants to alleviate or protect against these effects. This is an area where much additional research is needed.

Military research on occupational exposure to hazardous materials (hydraulic fluid, rocket motor propellants, etc.) has been done as a part of occupational health programs. Risks of exposure to chemical and biological warfare agents have increased as well as the potential for environmental warfare as was seen in the Persian Gulf. Deployments have become more frequent, and often into heavily polluted environments. Ozone and nitrogen dioxide are present in high concentrations in heavily polluted environments and can initiate free radical reactions that lead to lung damage. Studies in humans have shown protective effects of vitamin E against pollution damage. A study of 12 adult subjects evaluated the effects of daily vitamin E supplementation (600 mg) on red blood cell susceptibility to ozone-related free radical damage. Vitamin E significantly protected red blood cells at the highest levels of exposure, but not at lower levels of ozone exposure (Calabrese et al., 1985). However two other studies of Los Angeles residents exposed to photochemical smog showed no protective effect of vitamin E against short-term ozone exposure (Posin et al., 1979; Hackney et al., 1981). A triservice medical research and development program has begun to address some of these threats through a deployment toxicology research initiative, but no data are currently available in terms of nutritional strategies that would serve as protective mechanisms.

No data were available to assess the role of antioxidants in situations of hyperoxia, increased exposure to ionizing radiation, radiofrequency, UV light, and psychological stress. Studies of military personnel at high risk owing to their occupational duties are needed.

In conclusion, the limited data available suggest that supplementation for individuals exposed to multiple-stress situations associated with diminished food intake (e.g. Lower right hand shaded area of Figure 1) may be beneficial in maintaining intakes of antioxidants at or above the MRDA for those nutrients. An outcome monitoring component should be included as part of the overall health and environmental exposure activities since clear-cut evidence for efficacy of higher doses is not established.

3. Is there evidence of any health risk associated with supplemental intakes of Vitamin C, Vitamin E, or β-carotene by service members, taken with the intention of maintaining health and performance in adverse military training and operational environments?

The occurrence of adverse effects from consumption of large doses of vitamins C, E, and β-carotene appears to be low, however supplementation of these antioxidants is not without risk.

Vitamin C

Vitamin C intake in the range of 250-500 mg is very unlikely to cause adverse effects in the overwhelming majority of the population (Bendich, 1997). Possible exceptions would be individuals who form oxalates, and thus are prone to kidney stone formation (Chalmers et al., 1986).

A number of studies have been conducted on the effect of vitamin C intake on urinary oxalate excretion (Briggs, 1976; Hatch et al., 1980; Hughes et al., 1981; Fituri et al., 1983; Tsao et al., 1984). Daily doses have ranged from 1 to 10 grams. Findings have been conflicting, with some studies reporting no effects and others reporting large increases in urinary oxalate. Conflicting results may be explained in part by methodological problems in oxalate measurement since the presence of vitamin C in the urine interferes with urinary oxalate assays. No evidence clearly linking kidney stone formation to excess vitamin C intake was found (Curhan et al., 1996).

Other individuals who may be at risk include those who have iron storage diseases such as hereditary hemochromatosis or severe thalassemias. However the scientific basis for risk in these latter groups has not been firmly established (Bendich and Cohen, 1990). In the case of hereditary hemochromatosis it seems logical that increased consumption of vitamin C might increase the absorption of iron, but data are lacking on what the extent and impact of such an increase would be. Unfortunately the clinical manifestations of the disease are often not detected until middle age. In the case of severe thalassemias such as β-Thalassemia Major most of the increase in body iron is derived from repeated transfusions over a number of years and thus increased iron absorption is not considered to be the main cause of the iron overload. *In vitro* studies have shown that Vitamin C reduces unbound ferric iron, which in turn generates hydroxyl free radicals (Elsayed, 1997). However, virtually all iron in biological systems is in a bound state and not susceptible to this type of reaction.

There may be other potential risks. Results of one study suggested that 3 g of vitamin C per day for 6 days reduced high-altitude resistance in normal adults (Schrauzer et al., 1975). Other studies have indicated evidence of systemic conditioning (the accelerated metabolism of ascorbic acid) following abrupt discontinuation of prolonged, high dose vitamin C supplementation (Omaye et al., 1986, Schrauzer and Rhead, 1973; Tsao and Leung, 1988).

Recent research conducted at the National Institutes of Health (NIH) indicated that daily intakes of 100 mg of vitamin C saturated circulating immune cells and that this is reflective of other tissues in the body. Bioavailability of oral doses of vitamin C up to 200 mg was found to be 80%. Above that level, bioavailability declined rapidly. Consumption of vitamin C above 500 mg results in steady state conditions, the entire absorbed dose being excreted (Levine et al., 1996).

Although supplementation of up to 500 mg of vitamin C per day appears to pose little risk, data also indicate there is little benefit in providing supplements in excess of the 100 mg per day required for tissue and enzyme system saturation.

Vitamin E

Widely varying doses of vitamin E have been evaluated in numerous studies. In the α-Tocopherol, β-Carotene Cancer Prevention studies (ATBC Study Group, 1994) where subjects were given 50 mg tocopherol equivalents daily for 5 to 8 years, there was an increased risk of hemorrhagic stroke in the groups receiving vitamin E. The age of these subjects ranged from 50 to 69 yr. which is, on average, older than that of the military population. In a smaller study reported by Steiner et al. (1995), patients at high risk of stroke (as shown by transient ischemic attacks (TIA) and other transient neurologic deficits which often predate the occurrence of major strokes) were given 400 mg vitamin E plus aspirin for 2 years. Hemorrhagic stroke occurred in 2 of the 50 patients receiving vitamin E plus aspirin, while none were reported for those receiving aspirin only, although according to the investigator, this was not of statistical significance. Nevertheless it should be pointed out that the study population was selected on the basis of a tendency to form small blood clots in that they all had TIA and were therefore not likely to be classified as bleeders.

Individuals being treated with coumarin or Warfarin drugs have been reported to be at increased risk of hemorrhage if taking high doses of vitamin E (Corrigan and Ulfers, 1981). Jandak et al (1988) reported a significant reduction in platelet adhesion in healthy adults given 400 mg of d-α-tocopherol per day for 2 wk. Similar adverse effects have not been reported in other studies in healthy subjects given supplements of vitamin E as high as 800 mg to 1200 mg per day (Stampfer et al., 1988; Kitagawa and Mino, 1989; Kim and White, 1996).

Thus, supplements of vitamin E may pose a minor risk for the military population. Individuals routinely ingesting non-steroidal anti-inflammatory drugs such as aspirin, and anticoagulants may be at risk if supplemented with more than 50 mg of vitamin E.

Data supplied to the committee from Fort Hood, Texas, which houses 41,500 active duty soldiers, indicated that in 1997 44 % of soldiers were taking anti-inflammatory drugs, primarily ibuprofen, naprosyn, piroxicam, and aspirin, and that this estimate was considered to be a very conservative one (MAJ Vicky Thomas, Office of the Surgeon General, personal communication, September 22, 1998). Additional research is needed to define better any potential risk of vitamin E supplementation for those individuals who may be routinely consuming non-steroidal inflammatory drugs or anticoagulants. Concerns with respect to prolonged clotting times would be magnified in battlefield situations.

Beta Carotene

Carotenoids are widely distributed in fruits and vegetables with β-carotene being the most prevalent. For many years nutritionists have regarded high intakes of β-carotene as being innocuous and having no adverse effects other than causing skin discoloration. More recently, there have been a number of adverse effects of high levels of β-carotene reported in the scientific literature that would be of concern to military personnel.

Several reports have addressed the occurrence of amenorrhea associated with high intakes of β-carotene from fruits and vegetables (Duester et al., 1986; Frumar et al., 1979; Kemmann et al., 1983). Another study reported an interaction of ethanol with β-carotene causing delayed blood clearance of ethanol and enhanced hepatotoxicity (Leo et al., 1992).

Two recent prospective intervention trials designed to test the hypothesis that β-carotene might have a favorable chemopreventive effect against lung cancer in smokers revealed unexpected results (ATBC Study Group, 1994; Omenn et al., 1996a, b). In the ATBC trial, with a total of 29,133 male smokers, participants receiving β-carotene (20 mg per day alone, or in combination with 50mg of α-tocopherol) had an 18% increase in lung cancer and an 8% increase in mortality. In the Carotene and Retinol Efficacy Trial (CARET) (Omenn et al., 1996a, b) involving 18, 314 smokers and asbestos workers, 30 mg of β-carotene plus 25000 IU of retinol per day increased lung cancer incidence by 28% and mortality by 17%. However, in the Physicians Health Study, which included both smokers and non-smokers, no adverse effects of β-carotene were observed, nor were any benefits observed (Hennekens et al., 1996). In one long term study, Chinese subjects who were deficient in vitamin A received approximately 15 mg β-carotene daily, risk of stomach cancer decreased with no evidence of adverse effects (Blot et al., 1993). Several shorter studies with 25-90 mg of β-carotene per day showed positive effects in treating oral pre-malignant lesions, with no adverse side effects (Stich et al., 1988; Garewal et al., 1995).

The evidence suggests there may be an adverse effect of high doses of supplemental β-carotene in current heavy smokers and asbestos-exposed populations. Very recent data obtained using ferrets has demonstrated a plausible mechanism of β-carotene interaction with tobacco smoke that enhances lung tumor development (Wang et. al., 1999).

In view of these data, the committee does not recommend supplementation of β- carotene, even in high stress situations, especially since self-report data from the 1995 DoD World-wide Health Survey indicates that across all services (Army, Navy, Air Force, and Marines) 34% of males and 28% of females are smokers. Broken down by age group, 41% of males and 31% of females in the 18-25 age group are smokers. In addition, in the 18-25 age group (again by self-report which probably under-reports true incidence), 28.1% of males and 7.7% of females are heavy alcohol drinkers (defined as consuming 5 or more drinks in one day, at least one day per week).

It would appear that significant improvements in health status of military personnel could best be achieved through the promotion of healthy life-style changes.

REFERENCES

Alessio, H.M. and Goldfarb, A.H. 1988. Lipid peroxidation and scavenger enzymes during exercise: adaptive response to training. J. Appl. Physiol. 64:1333-1336.

Askew, E.W. 1995. Environmental and physical stress and nutrient requirements. Am. J. Clin. Nutr. 61(suppl):631S-637S.

ATBC (α-Tocopherol, β-carotene Cancer Prevention Study Group). 1994. The effect of vitamin E and β-carotene on the incidence of lung cancer and other cancers in male smokers. N. Engl. J. Med. 330:1029-1035.

Bendich, A. 1997. Vitamin C safety in humans. Pp. 367-379 in Vitamin C in Health and Disease. L. Packer and J. Fuchs (eds.). New York: Marcel Dekker, Inc.

Bendich, A. and Cohen, M. 1990. Ascorbic acid: Analysis of factors affecting iron absorption. Toxicology Lett.51:189-201

Bernton, E., D. Hoover, R. Galloway, and K. Popp. 1995. Adaptation to chronic stress in military trainees. Ann. NY. Acad. Sci. 774: 217-231.

Blot, W.J., J-Y. Li, P. R. Taylor, W. Guo, S. Dawsey, G.-Q. Wang, C.S. Yang, S.-F. Zheng, M. Gail, G.-Y. Li, Y. Yu, B.-Q. Lin, J. Tangrea, Y.-H. Sun, F. Liu, J.F. Fraumani, Jr., Y.-H. Zhang, and B. Li. 1993. Nutrition intervention trials in Linxian, China: Supplementation with specific vitamin/mineral combinations, cancer incidence, and disease-specific mortality in the general population. J. Natl. Cancer Inst. 85:1483-1491.

Briggs, M. 1976. Letter: Vitamin C-induced hyperoxaluria. Lancet I:154.

Calabrese, E.J., J. Victor, and M.A. Stoddard. 1985. Influence of dietary vitamin E on susceptibility to ozone exposure. Bull. Environ. Contam.Toxicol. 34:417-422.

Chalmers, A.H., D.M. Crowley and J.M. Brown. 1986. A possible etiological role for ascorbate in calculi formation. Clin. Chem. 32:333.

Clarkson, P.M. 1993. The effect of exercise and heat on vitamin requirements. In Nutritional Needs in Hot Environments pp.137-171. B. Marriott (ed.). Washington, D.C.: National Academy Press.

Collins, A.R., M. Dusinska, C.M. Gedik, and R. Stetina. 1996. Oxidative Damage to DNA: do we have a reliable biomarker. Environ. Health. Perspect. 104:465-469.

Corrigan, J.J., Jr., and L.L. Ulfers. 1981. Effect of vitamin E on prothrombin levels in warfarin-induced vitamin K deficiency. Am. J. Clin. Nutr. 34:1701-1705.

Curhan, G.C., W.C. Willett, E.B. Rimm and M.J. Stampfer. 1996. A prospective study of the intakes of vitamins C and B₆, and the risk of kidney stones in men. J. Urol. 155:1847-1851.

Davanipour, Z., E. Sobel, J.D. Bowman, Z. Qian, A.D. Will. 1997. Amyotrophic lateral sclerosis and occupational exposure to electromagnetic fields. Bioelectromagnetics 18:28-35.

Deuster, P.A., S.B. Kyle, P.B. Moser, R.A. Vigersky, A. Singh, E.B. Schoomaker. 1986. Nutritional intakes and status of highly trained amenorrheic and eumenorrheic women runners. Fertil. Steril. 46: 636-643.

DHHS (Department of Health and Human Services). 1991. Healthy People 2000: National Health Promotion and Disease Prevention Objectives. DHHS Publication No. (PHS) 91-50213. Washington, D.C.: U.S. Government Printing Office.

Elsayed, N.M., N.V. Gorbunov, V.E. Kagan. 1997. A proposed biochemical mechanism involving hemoglobin for blast overpressure-induced injury. Toxicol. 121:81-90.

Elsayed, N.M. 1997. Toxicology of blast overpressure. Toxicol. 121:1-15.

Fituri, N., N. Allawi, M. Bentley, and J. Costello. 1983. Urinary plasma oxalate during ingestion of pure ascorbic acid: A re-evaluation. Eur. Urol. 9:312-315.

Francis, K.T. and T. Hoobler. 1986. Failure of vitamin E and delayed muscle soreness. Alabama Medicine, J. of MASA. March, 1986 15-18.

Frumar, A.M., D.R. Meldrum, and H.L. Judd. 1979. Hypercarotenemia in hypothalamic amenorrhea. Fert. Steril. 32:261-264.

Garewal, H., F. Meyskens, R.V. Katz, 1995. β-carotene produces sustained remissions in oral leukoplakia: results of a 1 year randomized, controlled trial. Proc. Am. Soc. Clin. Oncol. (Abstract) 14:496.

Grayson, J.K. 1996. Radiation exposure, socioeconomic status and brain tumor risk in the U.S. Air Force: A nested case control study. Am. J. Epidemiol 143:480-486.

Gunnarsson, L.G., L. Bodin, B. Søderfeldt, O. Axelson. 1992. A case-control study of motor neuron disease: Its relation to heritability, and occupational exposures, particularly solvents. Br. J. Ind. Med. 49:791-798.

Hackney, J.D. W.S. Linn, R.D. Buckley, M.P. Jones, L.H. Wightman, S.K. Karuza, R.L. Blesseg, and H.J. Hislop. 1981. Vitamin E supplementation and respiratory effects of ozone in humans. J. Toxicol. Environ. Health. 7:383-390

Hatch, M., S. Mulgrew, E. Bourke, B. Keogh, and J. Costello. 1980. Effect of megadoses of ascorbic acid on serum and urinary oxalate. Eur. Urol. 6:166-169.

Hammeren, J., S. Powers, J. Lawler, D. Criswell, D. Lowenthal, and M. Pollack. 1993. Exercise training-induced alterations in skeletal muscle oxidative and antioxidant enzyme activity. Internat. J. Sports Med. 13: 412-416.

Hartmann, A., A.M. Nieb, M. Grunert-Fuchs, B. Poch, and G.Speit. 1995. Vitamin E prevents exercise-induced DNA damage. Mutation Res. 346:195-202.

Hennekens, C.H. 1998. Antioxidant Vitamins: Current and Future Directions. Presented at IOM Workshop: *Antioxidants and the Effects of Oxidative Stress in Military Personnel.* July 30, 1998. Washington, D.C.

Hennekens, C.H., J.E. Buring, J.E. Manson, M. Stampfer, B. Rosner, N.R. Cook, C.Belanger, F. LaMotte, J.M. Gaziano, P.M. Ridker, W. Willett, and R. Peto. 1996. Lack of effect of long-term supplementation of beta carotene on the incidence of malignant neoplasms and cardiovascular disease. New Engl. J. Med. 334:1145-1149.

Hornig, D.H., U. Moser, B.E. Glatthaar. 1988. Ascorbic acid. Pp. 417-435 in Modern Nutrition in Health and Disease. 7th Edition. M.E. Shils and V.R. Young (eds.). Philadelphia: Lea & Febiger.

Hughes, C. S. Dutton, A.S. Truswell. 1981. High intakes of ascorbic acid and urinary oxalate. J. Hum. Nutr. 35:274.

IOM (Institute of Medicine). 1993. Nutritional Needs in Hot Environments. B. Marriott (ed.). Washington, D.C.: National Academy Press.

IOM. 1995. Not Eating Enough. B. Marriott (ed.). Washington D.C.: National Academy Press

IOM. 1998. Military Strategies for Sustainment of Nutrition and Immune Function in the Field. Washington, D.C: National Academy Press

IOM. 1996. Nutritional Needs in Cold and High Altitude Environments. B. Marriott and S.J. Carlson (eds.). Washington, D.C. National Academy Press.

Jacob, R.A. 1994. Vitamin C. Pp. 432-448 in Modern Nutrition in Health and Disease. 8th Edition. M.E. Shils, J. A. Olson, and M. Shike (eds.) Philadelphia, PA: Lea & Febiger.

Jakeman, P. and S. Maxwell. 1993. Effect of antioxidant vitamin supplementation on muscle function after eccentric exercise. Eur. J. Appl. Physiol. 67:426-430

Jandak, J., M. Steiner, and P.D. Richardson. 1988. Reduction of platelet adhesiveness by vitamin E supplementation in humans. Thromb. Res. 49:393-404.

Janero, D.R. 1990. Malondialdehyde and thiobarturic acid-reactivity as diagnostic indices of lipid peroxidation and peroxidative tissue damage. Free Radic. Biol. Med. 9:515-540.

Kantner, M. 1998. Free radicals, exercise and antioxidant supplementation. Proc. Nutr. Soc. 57:9-13.

Kemmann, E., S.A. Pasquale, and R.Skaf. 1983. Amenorrhea associated with carotenemia. J. Am. Med. Assoc. 249:926-929.

Kim, J.M., and R.H. White. 1996. Effect of vitamin E on the anticoagulant response to warfarin. Am. J. Cardiol. 77:545-546.

Kitagawa, M. and M. Mino. 1989. Effects of elevated d-alpha-tocopherol dosages in man. J. Nutr. Sci. Vitaminol. (Tokyo) 35:133-142.

Lawrence, J.D., R.C. Bower, W.P.Riehl, and J.L. Smith. 1975. Effects of alpha-tocopherol acetate on the swimming endurance of trained swimmers. Am. J. Clin. Nutr. 28:205-208.

Leo, M.A., C. Kim, N. Lowe, and C.S. Lieber. 1992. Interaction of ethanol with beta-carotene: delayed blood clearance and enhanced hepatotoxicity. Hepatology 15:883-891.

Levine, M., C. Conry-Cantilena, Y. Wang, R.W. Welch, P.W. Washko, K.R. Dhariwal, J.B. Park, A. Lazarev, J.F. Graumlich, J. King, and L.R. Cantilena. 1996. Vitamin C pharmacokinetics in healthy volunteers: evidence for a recommended dietary allowance. Proc. Natl. Acad. Sci. USA 93:3704-3709.

Meydani, M., W.J. Evans, G. Handelman, L. Biddle, R.A. Fielding, S.N. Meydani, J. Burrill, M.A. Fiatarone, J.B. Blumburg, and J.G. Cannon. 1993. Protective effect of vitamin E on exercise-induced oxidative damage in young and older adults. Am. J. Physiol. 264:R992-R998.

Moore, R.J., K.E. Friedl, T.R. Kramer, L.E. Martinez-Lopez, R.W. Hoyt, R.T. Tulley, J.P. DeLany, E.W. Askew, and J.A. Vogel. 1992. Changes in soldier nutritional status and immune function during the Ranger training course. Technical Report T13-92. Natick, MA: U.S. Army Research Institute of Environmental Medicine.

NRC (National Research Council). 1989. Diet and Health: Implications for Reducing Chronic Disease Risk. Washington, D.C.: National Academy Press.

Omaye, S.T., J.H. Skala, R.A. Jacob. 1986. Plasma ascorbic acid in adult males: Effects of depletion and supplementation. Am. J. Clin. Nutr. 44:257-264.

Omenn, G.S., G.E. Goodman, M.D. Thornquist, J. Balmes, M.R. Cullen, A. Glass, J.P. Keogh, F.L. Meyskens, B. Valanis, J.H. Williams, S. Barnhart, and S. Hammar. 1996(a). Effects of a combination of beta carotene and vitamin A on lung cancer and cardiovascular disease. New Engl. J. Med. 334:1150-1155.

Omenn, G.S., G.E. Goodman, M.D. Thornquist, J. Balmes, M.R. Cullen, A. Glass, J.P. Keogh, F.L. Meyskens, B. Valanis, J.H. Williams, S. Barnhart, and S. Hammar. 1996(b). Risk factors for lung cancer and for intervention effects in CARET, the Beta-Carotene and Retinol Efficacy Trial. J. Natl. Cancer Inst. 88:1550-1559.

Patrono, C., and G.A. Fitzgerald. 1997. Isoprostanes: potential markers of oxidative stress in artherothrombotic disease. Arterioscler. Thromb. Vasc. Biol. 17: 2309-2315.

Posin, C.I., K.W. Clark, M/P/ Jones, R.D. Buckley, and J.D. Hackney. 1979. Human biochemical response to ozone and vitamin E. J. Toxicol. Environ. Health. V:1049-1058.

Reynolds, R.D. 1996. Effects of cold and altitude on vitamin and mineral requirements. Pp. 215-244 in Nutritional Needs in Cold and High Altitude Environments B.M. Marriott and S.J. Carlson, eds.. IOM. Washington D.C.: National Academy Press.

Reynolds, K.L., H. A. Heckel, C.E. Witt, J.N. Martin, J.A. Pollard, J.J. Knapick, and B.H. Jones. 1994. Cigarette smoking, physical fitness, and injuries in infantry soldiers. Am. J. Prev. Med. 10:145-150.

Rokitzki, L., E. Logemann, G. Huber, E. Keck, and J. Keul. 1994. Alpha-tocopherol supplementation in racing cyclists during extreme endurance training. Int. J. Sports Nutr. 4:253-264.

Schrauzer, G.N., D. Ishmael, and G.W. Kiefer. 1975. Some aspects of current vitamin C usage: Diminished high-altitude resistance following overdosage. Ann. NY Acad. Sci. 258:377-381.

Schrauzer, G.N. and W.J. Rhead. 1973. Ascorbic acid abuse: Effects of long-term ingestion of excessive amounts on blood levels and urinary excretion. Int. J. Vit. Nutr. Res. 43: 201-211.

Seis, H. 1986. Biochemistry of oxidative stress. Angew. Chem. Int. Ed. Engl. 25:1058-1071.

Sen, C.K., 1995. Oxidants and antioxidants in exercise. J. Appl. Physiol. 79:675-686.

Sen, C.K., M. Atalay, and O. Hanninen. 1994. Exercise induced oxidative stress: Glutathione supplementation and deficiency J. Applied Physiol. 77: 2177-2187.

Sharman, I.M., M.G. Down, and N.G. Norgan. 1976. The effects of vitamin E on physiological function and athletic performance of trained swimmers. J. Sports Med. 16:215-225.

Shippee, R., K. Friedl, T. Kramer, M. Mays, K. Popp, E.W. Askew, B. Fairbrother, R. , J. Vogel, L. Marchitelli, P. Frykman, L. Martinez-Lopez, E. Bernton, M. Kramer, R. Tulley, J. Rood, J. Delany, D. Jezior, and J. Arsenault. 1994. Nutritional and immunological assessment of Ranger students with increased caloric intake. Technical Report T95-5. Natick, MA: U.S. Army Research Institute of Environmental Medicine.

Simon-Schnass, I. 1996. Oxidative stress at high altitudes and effects of vitamin E. Pp. 393-418 in Nutritional Needs in Cold and High Altitude Environments. B. Marriott and S.J. Carlson, eds.. IOM. Washington D.C.: National Academy Press

Simon-Schnass, I. and H. Pabst. 1988. Influence of vitamin E on physical performance. Internat. J. Vit. Nutr. Res. 58:49-54.

Sobel, E., Z. Davanipour, R. Suldava, T. Erkinjuntti, J. Wikstrom, V.W. Henderson, G. Buckwalter, J.D. Bowman, P.J. Lee. 1995. Occupations with exposure to electromagnetic fields: A possible risk factor for Alzheimer's disease. Am. J. Epidemiol. 142:515-524.

Sobel, E., M. Dunn, Z. Davanipour, Z. Qian, H.C. Chui. 1996. Elevated risk of Alzheimer's disease among workers with likely electromagnetic field exposure. Neurology 47:1477-1481.

Stampfer, M.J., J.A. Jakubowski, D. Faigel, R. Vaillancourt, and D. Deykin. 1988. Vitamin E supplementation effect on human platelet function, arachidonic acid metabolism, and plasma prostacyclin levels. Am. J. Clin. Nutr. 47:700-706.

Steiner, M. 1991. Influence of vitamin E on platelet function in humans. J. Am. Coll. Nutr. 10:466-473.

Stich, H.F., M.P. Rosin, P. Hornby, B. Matthew, R. Sankaranarayanan, M.K. Nair. 1988. Remission of oral leukoplakias and micronuclei in tobacco/betel quid chewers treated with β-carotene and with β-carotene plus vitamin A. Int. J. Cancer 42:195

Tsao, C.S. and P.Y. Leung. 1988. Urinary ascorbic acid levels following the withdrawal of large doses of ascorbic acid in guinea pigs. J. Nutr. 118:895-900.

Tsao, C.S., and S.L. Salimi. 1984. Effect of large intake of ascorbic acid on urinary and plasma oxalic acid levels. Int. J. Vit. Nutr. Res. 54:245.

USDA (U.S. Department of Agriculture) and DHHS. 1995. Nutrition and Your Health: Dietary Guidelines for Americans, Fourth Edition. Home and Garden Bulletin No. 232. Washington, D.C.: U.S. Government Printing Office

Wang, X-D., C. Liu, R.T. Broderick, D.E. Smith, N.I. Krinsky, and R.M. Russell. 1999. Retinoid signaling and activator protein-1 expression in ferrets given β-carotene supplements and exposed to tobacco smoke. J. Nat. Cancer Inst. 91:60-66.

Antioxidants and Oxidative Stress in Military Personnel

July 29-31, 1998
National Academy of Sciences
2101 Constitution Avenue, N.W.
Washington, D.C. 20418

WORKSHOP PARTICIPANTS

CMNR
Robert Nesheim
Salinas, CA

Lawrence E. Armstrong Ph.D.
Professor, Departments of
  Physiology and Neurobiology,
  and Exercise Science
Human Performance Laboratory
University of Connecticut
Storrs, CT

William R. Beisel, M.D.
Adjunct Professor, Department of
  Molecular Microbiology and
  Immunology
The Johns Hopkins University
  School of Hygiene and Public
  Health
Baltimore, MD

Wanda Chenoweth, Ph.D., R.D.
Professor, Department of Food
  Science and Human Nutrition
Michigan State University
East Lansing, MI

Robin B. Kanarek, Ph.D.
Professor and Chair of Psychology
Professor of Nutrition
Tufts University
Medford, MA

Orville A. Levander, Ph.D.
Research Leader, Nutrient
  Requirements and Functions
  Laboratory
USDA-ARS Beltsville Human
  Nutrition Research Center
Beltsville, MD

Esther M. Sternberg, M.D.
Chief, Neuroendocrine
  Immunology and Behavior
National Institute of Mental Health-
  NIH
Bethesda, MD

John E. Vanderveen, Ph.D. ·
Rockville, MD

Douglas W. Wilmore, M.D.
Frank Sawyer Professor
Department of Surgery
Brigham and Women's Hospital
Boston, MA

Food and Nutrition Board Liaison
Johanna T. Dwyer, D.Sc., R.D.
Professor, Departments of
  Medicine and of Community
  Health
Tufts Medical School and School
  of Nutrition Science and Policy
Director, Frances Stern Nutrition
  Ctr., New England Medical Ctr.
Boston, MA

U.S. Army Grant Officer
Representative
LTC Karl Friedl, Ph.D.
Program Director
Army Operational Medicine
  Research
USAMRC
Fort Detrick, MD

Speakers
Eldon Wayne Askew, Ph.D.
Professor and Director
Division of Foods and Nutrition
University of Utah
Salt Lake City, UT

Lt. Gen. Ronald Blanck
Surgeon General, U.S. Army

Patrick Dunne, Ph.D.
U.S. Army Natick Research,
  Development, and Engineering
  Center
U.S. Army Soldier System
  Command
Natick, MA

Nabil M. Elsayed, Ph. D.
Chief, Pulmonary Biochemistry
  Section
Department of Respiratory
  Research
Division of Medicine
Walter Reed Army Institute of
  Research
Washington, D.C.

Hank Gardner, Ph.D.
Director
USARIEM
Fort Detrick, MD

Charles Hennekens, M.D., Ph.D.
Eugene Braunwald Professor of
  Medicine
Harvard Medical School
Chief, Div. of Preventive Medicine
Brigham and Womens Hospital
Boston, MA

MAJ William H. Karge, Ph.D.
Nutritional Biochemist
USARIEM
Natick, MA

Susan Taylor Mayne, Ph.D.
Associate Professor in Chronic
  Disease Epidemiology
Department of Epidemiology and
  Public Health
Yale University School of
  Medicine
New Haven, CT

Harold Schmitz, Ph.D.
Group Manager
M&M Mars Company
Hackettstown, NJ

Ronald L. Seaman, Ph.D.
Research Scientist
Microwave Bioeffects Branch,
USARMD
Brooks AFB, TX

Chandan K. Sen, Ph.D.
Staff Scientist
Biological Technologies Section
Lawrence Berkeley National
  Laboratory/EETD
University of California
Berkeley, CA

Maret G. Traber, Ph.D.
Principal Investigator, Linus
    Pauling Institute
Associate Professor, Dept. of
    Nutrition and Food Management
Oregon State University
Corvallis, OR

Steven Wood, Ph.D., R.D.
Senior Clinical Project Leader
Ross Products Division
Columbus, OH

FNB Staff
Mary Poos, Ph.D.
Sydne Newberry, Ph.D.
Melissa Van Doren
Allison Yates, Ph.D.

Appendix L

Conclusions and Recommendations from the Workshop Report Military Strategies for Sustainment of Nutrition and Immune Function in the Field

Submitted May 1999

Committee Responses to Questions, Conclusions, and Recommendations

COMMITTEE RESPONSES TO QUESTIONS

As stated in Chapter 1 of this report, the Committee on Military Nutrition Research was asked to review the state of knowledge concerning the impact of nutritional status on immune function. Below are the committee's answers to the five questions posed by the Army regarding nutrition and sustainment of immune function in the field, followed by the committees conclusions and recommendations. Recommendations for areas of future development for the U.S. Army nutrition research programs are also included.

1. What are the significant military hazards or operational settings most likely to compromise immune function in soldiers?

As described previously and outlined below, many conditions or stressors have been associated with compromised immune function during Ranger training and basic combat training, as well as during arctic training and in deployments to locations such as Somalia, Haiti, Panama, and the Persian Gulf.

• *Reduced ration consumption.* Intakes less than 60 percent of the total energy needed, particularly during exposure to harsh environments and/or dehydration, were shown to be a significant stressor. In U.S. Ranger II, the increase in energy intake from that in Ranger I (2,780 to 3,250 calories or approximately 470 kcal/d), which tempered weight loss to only 12.8 percent of initial body weight, appeared to minimize the adverse effects on immune function. Thus, weight loss, particularly that involving lean body mass, appears to be a major factor in inducing immune system dysfunction.

The effects of dehydration on immune function are not reviewed in this report. However, weight losses of as little as 3–5 percent in 24–48 h, which are primarily due to dehydration, have a significant impact on performance. Weight losses of 6–10 percent in a similar period may affect health adversely. Thus, the effects of dehydration must be separated from those of underconsumption of rations (see IOM, 1995).

• *Prolonged moderate-to-heavy physical activity.* The week-long Norwegian Ranger training studies with heavy exercise and limited sleep did not demonstrate significant weight loss or alterations in immune function, whereas the U.S. Ranger I study of 8- to 9-week duration demonstrated a greater weight loss (14 percent of body weight) and an altered immune response. Low- to moderate-intensity exercise (<60 percent $Vo_{2\,max}$), such as that performed in most troop activity of a duration of 60 minutes or less, appears to exert less stress on the immune system than activity that is more strenuous (>60 percent $Vo_{2\,max}$) performed for longer than 1 h. Repeated bouts of strenuous activity may increase the risk of infection, particularly of the upper respiratory tract.

• *Limited, interrupted or nonrestful sleep.* Limited or nonrestful sleep over a prolonged period (as little as 3 hours or less was noted in the Norwegian Ranger studies), particularly when coupled with stressful physical activity, may result in some compromise of the immune system. Short periods of severe caloric and sleep deprivation appear to have less adverse effect on immune function than a more prolonged period with greater weight loss (caloric deficit).

• *Increased infection and injury.* This category includes infections associated with trauma and burns, such as cellulitis, osteomyelitis, wound abscesses, and sepsis, as well as naturally occurring infections and diseases such as conjunctivitis, otitis, upper and lower respiratory tract infections, urinary tract infections, and gastroenteritis. Diarrhea is commonly experienced by soldiers in military operations, most likely due to exposure to infectious organisms from strange environments (dust, water, local foods). Influenza also is common, and in some environments, other diseases occur that are rare in the United States.

• *Increased exposure to extremes of temperature and humidity.* Increased exposures in areas such as the tropics or desert, as well as with operations in the arctic areas of North America or northern Europe during winter conditions, can adversely affect food intake and sleep. Heavy activity or environmental extremes may increase energy requirements by as much as 15 percent after acclimatization without compensatory ration intake. For example, hypohydration may lead to temporary anorexia and a worsening cycle of lowered water and food intake. The factors that influence ration consumption may be even more significant for operations in the cold and at high altitudes.

• *Increased psychological stresses.* Stresses such as those imposed by deployment, separation from family, imminence of combat, threat of biological agents, and long periods of vigilance with interrupted sleep and inadequate rest, may also be significant and often result in field training- or combat-induced anorexia. All of these factors may impinge on immunological health.

• *Prolonged exposure during training or battlefield combat to environmental assaults.* Environmental exposure (for example, to smoke or fumes from fuels or chemicals, dust, dirt, and blast overpressure) may induce oxidative stress on protective systems.

2. What methods for assessment of immune function are most appropriate in military nutrition laboratory research, and what methods are most appropriate for field research?

It is important first to identify a number of methodologic issues that must be considered when assessing immune function.

Technical Issues

In addition to the choice of assay, a large number of issues must be considered in the design of studies to assess immune function. The first consideration in a study of immune challenge is the choice of antigen, described previously for tests of primary and secondary antibody response (Cunningham-Rundles, 1999; Straight et al., 1994).

The second consideration is the timing of sample collection. As described by Erhard Haus (Chapter 20), the immune system is significantly influenced by biological rhythms; thus, samples must be drawn on an established schedule (Straight et al., 1994). Additionally, it is important to standardize collections in relation to physical activity because differential cell counts can change acutely during and immediately after exercise (DeRijk et al., 1996, 1997).

The third, and possibly most critical consideration, is the protocol for storage and transportation of samples. According to G. Sonnenfeld (University of Kentucky, Louisville, personal communication, 1997), human blood samples must be shipped at room temperature in Styrofoam containers, and for most status indicators, must be assayed within 24 h. If necessary, some preparatory steps, such as harvesting cells from blood, may be performed in rudimentary makeshift labs and the samples sent under controlled conditions to a central facility for completion of analysis.

A fourth but related consideration is the choice of laboratory for sample analysis. The Agency for Toxic Substances and Disease Registry (ATSDR) of the Department of Health and Human Services recommends the use of a central or core reference facility for all analyses to avoid small differences in protocols and solutions used. Some methods, such as the measurement of mitogen-induced lymphocyte proliferation by [^{3}H]thymidine incorporation are extremely sensitive to such factors (Cunningham-Rundles, Chapter 9). Thymidine incorporation is also a variable, relatively nonspecific measure not easily standardized and not well applicable to field studies. Because some procedures must be performed within a short period of time, the number of samples that can be processed is thus limited.

Finally, the use of controls is extremely critical both in the collection and assessment of samples and in the interpretation of data. It is recommended that each time samples are drawn and an assay is performed, a standard is drawn and included for the assay, consisting of the blood (or cells) of one individual, to correct for intraindividual and interassay variability. Whenever possible, subjects should be used as their own baselines, and longitudinal studies should be performed (Straight et al., 1994). Of major concern are the lack of population-based normative reference ranges for most immune function parameters and the need to obtain complete health histories (including such factors as smoking, use of other drugs, and pregnancy) from subjects to rule out possible confounding factors.

Methodologic Issues

Immunologic function can be related to nutritional status by utilizing two distinct methodological approaches. First, under *controlled* conditions, normal healthy individuals can be studied; after an appropriate baseline period, a nutritional perturbation can be imposed and the changes in immune responses from baseline determined. This approach allows single nutrient or environmental perturbations to be studied while many other factors that also cause immune dysfunction are controlled. In addition, appropriate controls (with adequate sample size) can be included, and a period of refeeding (or second control period) can be included at the end of the experiment.

Second, in *field* studies, the conditions are quite different, and other variables, in addition to altered nutritional intake, affect individuals. Immune dysfunction due to both nutritional and other operational stressors may be present. Under these conditions, it is possible to study the incidence of infection using epidemiologic techniques, while food intake and nutritional status are determined. Appropriate ambulatory tests of immunologic function can be validated and compared to results obtained in more controlled settings.

A longitudinal study of immune function in simulated combat conditions in the field could be performed that would have the ability to detect accurately over time the subjects' nutritional state and the incidence of infection. When clinical signs are clearly defined and documented, and symptoms indicate the occurrence of infectious illnesses, studies to determine etiology and therapy can be initiated, along with serial studies of C-reactive protein (CRP), erythrocyte sedimentation rate (ESR), acute-phase reactants, whole blood, plasma, cytokines, and their receptors. The longitudinal course of illness can then be correlated with nutritional parameters.

Prior to pursuing field investigations, researchers must undertake appropriate studies in a controlled clinical setting to answer some of the more basic questions about the impact of altered nutritional status on immune function. These studies must precede those that attempt to confer a state of enhanced immune function or to study the response to a specific nutrient. For example, limited studies of subjects placed under conditions of reduced caloric intake could be undertaken. Attempts could also be made to see if supplementation with one or more essential single nutrients could maintain normal immunological competence in the face of generalized dietary deprivation. Before extensive field evaluations of the influence of nutrition on immune response are undertaken, carefully controlled laboratory studies should be performed and data collected from more fundamental research studies. To hypothesize which of the nutrients may enhance immune response, it may be helpful first to determine under controlled conditions which nutrients, by their deficiency or exclusion from the diet, impact the immune response negatively; however, this will not provide a complete picture.

The CMNR confirms the need to determine appropriate field measures for monitoring the immune response, particularly for determining the presence and magnitude of an acute-phase reaction, which may be adversely influenced by nutritional status in stressed individuals. Based on standardized test panels recommended by government agencies or private-sector scientists, the committee suggests the following. If clinical signs of infection are present or there has been significant weight loss induced by nutritional stress, a simple-to-use basic screening panel of immune function tests such as CRP protein, ESR, a baseline battery (testing six or more antibody titers for several previously administered military vaccines, immunoglobulins G, A, and M; and complete blood count with CD4 lymphocyte count and CD4:CD8 ratio should be employed initially. In the event that these basic tests of immune response indicate the existence of immune compromise of an unusual nature or unusually great incidence, the CMNR suggests a second tier of immune function tests. These would include natural killer (NK) cell numbers and activities; lymphocyte mitogenesis assays; thymosin measurements; and estimations of phagocytic cell chemotaxis and microbicidal activities (for example, *Listeria monocytogenes*-killing assay). However, these tests must first be validated for field use. A standardized battery of delayed dermal hypersensitivity tests may be employed at baseline and again if stress-induced weight loss exceeds 10 percent.

If validated, these tests would be valuable in research studies for rapid field assessment of immune status and might suggest steps that could be taken to improve resistance to potential exposures and thus improve unit effectiveness. As previously noted by the CMNR (IOM, 1997), tests based on cytokine assays, especially of the proinflammatory cytokines and related molecules excreted in urine and whole-blood cytokine production assays, have great potential for adding important new diagnostic measures at a relatively low cost–benefit ratio.

Differential changes in production patterns of specific cytokines (that is., shifts from T-helper 1 [Th1] to Th2-type patterns) may be the most sensitive way to determine whether changes in immune responses are stress related. Such tests currently are being evaluated in many civilian research studies and may have very real potential value for suggesting the presence of cytokine-induced malnutrition in military personnel who are being exposed to the stresses of rigorous training exercises or ongoing operational missions. Additionally, in the development and validation of more precise readout measures, attention should be paid to the development of microassays that can be applied in field settings to minimize stress and blood loss during sampling.

3. The proinflammatory cytokines have been proposed to decrease lean body mass, mediate thermoregulatory mechanisms, and increase resistance to infectious disease by reducing metabolic activity in a way that is similar to the reduction seen in malnutrition and other catabolic conditions. Interventions to sustain immune function can alter the actions, nutritional costs, and potential changes in the levels of proinflammatory cytokines. What are the benefits and risks to soldiers of such interventions?

One of the most fundamental needs is to sustain the functional competence of the immune system in military personnel who must experience the stresses of rigorous training and operational assignments and who face the risks of infectious illnesses as well as diverse forms of trauma. Cytokine effects in the body can be influenced by a variety of factors as outlined below.

• *Nutritional interventions.* It is well known that in the course of infection, proinflammatory cytokines mediate the loss of specific nutrients, which must be repleted or redistributed. In turn, growing evidence suggests that a number of nutrients may influence immune function by affecting synthesis of specific cytokines, their soluble receptors, or inhibitory factors. For example, research on the antioxidant vitamins A, E, and C, as well as certain polyunsaturated fatty acids (PUFAs) and amino acids (AAs), has shown that their apparent ability to modulate immune status may be mediated by their effects on cytokines, at least under some conditions, but many questions remain regarding the efficacy of these nutrients in amounts that exceed Military Recommended Dietary Allowance (MRDA) levels. Research is also needed on whether nutritional intervention during stress is effective or whether it must be combined with agents that suppress inflammation.

• *Pharmacological interventions (including immunizations).* Research has demonstrated that a number of pharmacological agents including aspirin, ibuprofen, and glucocorticoids modulate the effects of cytokines and can be used to minimize signs and symptoms of cytokine-induced acute-phase reactions and the nutrient losses that accompany them. Glucocorticoids can block fever and reduce many of the metabolic consequences of acute-phase responses caused when proinflammatory cytokines are released by cells, but the adverse consequences of prolonged systemic administration of glucocorticoids have long been recognized. On the other hand, drugs such as aspirin and ibuprofen can block the intracellular formation of many of the eicosanoids (prostaglandins, prostacyclins, leukotrienes, thromboxanes) and thereby reduce the fevers, myalgias, and headaches that accompany cytokine-induced acute-phase reactions. Because losses of body nutrients during these reactions are often proportional to the magnitude and duration of fevers, the use of such generally safe and effective anti-inflammatory drugs serves indirectly to maintain the body's nutritional status and immune system functions. Further, the use of anti-inflammatory drugs for the management of minor traumas or infections (for example, upper respiratory tract infections) is well recognized and provides for sustained military performance during severe training exercises and operational missions. The immune system can be "educated" in advance by the prophylactic administration of immunizations against all possible foreign agents. Such immunization procedures do carry some risks, depending on the vaccine being administered, but the ultimate military benefits of such immunization practices far outweigh the risks. Furthermore, the risks of immunization can be reduced and the benefits increased (that is, improved vaccine effectiveness) by the use of oral vaccines, whose development by the military was recommended in an earlier CMNR report (IOM, 1997).

• *Administration of products of biotechnology.* Biotechnological methods have allowed the production of many individual cytokines and their receptors. At the present time, their use is limited to the administration of granulocyte macrophage colony stimulating factor for the treatment of bone marrow recipients and those undergoing a limited number of other experimental procedures, and their effectiveness has not been demonstrated in healthy subjects or in clinical trials. A recent review by Mackowiak and colleagues (1997) discusses the therapeutic use of pyrogenic cytokines and the use of their inhibitors. The authors comment on the failure, or even the harm, associated with their therapeutic use in humans (in contrast to rodents). The administration of exogenous cytokines and the modulation of cytokines in vivo are areas of active research in the civilian sector; the use of cytokines to enhance resistance to infections, however, should be carefully studied in animals before application to clinical situations.

4. What are the important safety and regulatory considerations in the testing and use of nutrients or dietary supplements to sustain immune function under field conditions?

The basic considerations in the testing and fielding of nutrients or dietary supplements to sustain immune function are to ensure, first, that the nutrients are in fact safe under the conditions of intended use and, second, that they are effective. Since the levels of some of the nutrients that must be fed to achieve potential effects are much higher than levels usually ingested in foods, further safety testing is warranted. Such testing involves attempts to delineate the upper limits of safety.

For any substance, there are a number of major considerations relevant to the question posed. These include the following:

- the intake levels that are suggested and referenced by the Recommended Dietary Allowance (RDA)/MRDA;
  - the customary range of intake;
  - the tolerable upper level;
  - the safety and efficacy of the substance at the level of intended use; and
  - special groups or circumstances that deserve attention.

Generally accepted tolerable upper intake limit values have not yet been established for individual nutrients, but the Food and Nutrition Board's (FNB's) Subcommittee on Upper Reference Levels of Nutrients is now considering these levels. For purposes of planning further military research on individual nutrients, there is already evidence that safety problems associated with excess consumption are much more likely for some nutrients than for others. In clinical practice, the general rule of thumb is that it is generally unwise to exceed three to four times the traditional RDA for most fat-soluble vitamins; however, margins of safety may be lower for vitamins A and D in some groups. In general, water-soluble vitamins tend to be less toxic and can be consumed in larger multiples of the traditional RDA than can fat-soluble vitamins.

Trace minerals are difficult to discuss in general terms. It is important to remember that supplements of a single nutrient cannot be considered in isolation. The World Health Organization (WHO, 1996) Expert Consultation examined upper safe levels for trace minerals and concluded that the toxicity and the potential for nutrient–nutrient interactions must be considered individually. Risks of pathology resulting from such interactions are higher when intakes of other essential nutrients with which they interact are low or marginal, accentuating the nutrient imbalance. Therefore, conservatism is warranted in the consumption of trace minerals in excess of traditional RDA or suggested safe and adequate levels. However, requirements may change during an episode of illness, and requirements for some minerals may substantially increase (for example, zinc during diarrhea). The FNB's Dietary Reference

Intakes (DRIs) Subcommittee on Upper Safe Levels is now considering the issue more fully.

Dietary deficiencies of a variety of nutritionally essential trace elements (zinc, copper, selenium) have been demonstrated to have an adverse impact on immune function in laboratory animals and elderly humans, and deficiencies of zinc and copper have resulted in increased susceptibility to certain infections in humans. Excessive intakes of some trace elements have led to immuno-suppressive effects. Therefore, care must be exercised in the use of single-nutrient supplements until the optimal range of intakes for these trace elements is determined.

Iron. Both iron deficiency and iron excess appear to have the potential to increase susceptibility to infection. In a military situation, it is likely that the potential reduction in immune function due to iron deficiency is of more significance than any effects of iron overload. Because of their higher iron requirement and lower intake of operational rations, the iron intake of female soldiers may be lower than recommended in the MRDA, increasing their risk for iron deficiency anemia. Utilizing as the criterion for iron deficiency a serum ferritin concentration of less than 12 µg/L, and a combination of low serum ferritin and a hemoglobin of less than 120 g/L as the criteria for iron deficiency anemia, it was shown that 17 percent of new female recruits entering basic combat training (BCT) fit these criteria for iron deficiency, while 8 percent could be classified as having iron deficiency anemias. A survey of a similar (but not the same) population of women at the end of BCT showed that by the end of training, 33 percent were iron deficient and 26 percent were anemic (Westphal et al., 1994, 1995).

Iron deficiency anemia can be expected to have adverse effects on the military performance of both men and women depending in part on its severity. Performance deficits in both men and women due to compromised iron status have been demonstrated most clearly during exercise of prolonged duration, such as long-distance running (Newhouse and Clement, 1988). Iron deficiency anemia may also have an adverse impact on recovery from serious wounds or injuries, especially those that involve large amounts of blood loss. However, data to support deficits in physical performance in iron-compromised individuals have not been systematically collected by the military. Some preliminary evidence suggests that iron supplementation of nonanemic women can improve aerobic capacity (J. Haas, Cornell University, personal communication, 1977). Male soldiers consuming operational rations appear to meet iron needs, as judged from current levels in the MRDA.

Glutamine. Glutamine is an amino acid that constitutes approximately 5 percent of most proteins. The CMNR recognizes that glutamine is a potential candidate for addition to operational rations to optimize immunity. It has demonstrated potential for promoting immune cell proliferation and improving immune function, especially under the stress of surgery, infection, or bowel disease. However, before it would be appropriate to consider providing supplemental glutamine to soldiers in training or deployment situations, it will first be necessary to demonstrate in a healthy population the benefits of providing glutamine at levels significantly greater than those normally obtained in the diet. The results of one military study presented at the workshop showed no beneficial effects of glutamine supplementation on immune function parameters. The CMNR recently hosted a workshop (The Role of Protein and Amino Acids in Sustaining and Enhancing Performance) that addressed more fully the safety and efficacy issues for this and other amino acids.

Vitamin A and Antioxidants. Vitamin A intakes beyond the MRDA do not appear to be beneficial; in fact, excess intakes can be toxic. Healthy adult men and women of military age represent the lowest-risk group for the development of vitamin A deficiency; however, under certain conditions, such as chronic infection or prolonged dietary deprivation, the risk of vitamin A deficiency and associated immune abnormalities may be significant (Semba, Chapter 12). Carotenoids as supplied from fruits and vegetables may be important as modulators or stimulators of immune function.

Vitamins C and E are immunopotentiating agents most likely because of their function as antioxidants. Both of these vitamins are relatively nontoxic. However, it has not been demonstrated whether there is a functional benefit of increased intakes in protection against cancer, pathogenic viruses, or bacteria. Investigation of the role of these vitamins in protecting against or modulating the effects of infection is an active area of research. Toxicities of high-dose vitamin C supplements also have been difficult to demonstrate. Some evidence suggests that doses of 500 mg or more may result in increased excretion of oxalate (a precursor to one form of renal stone), but this observation has been limited to individuals who have an increased risk of forming stones (Urivetsky et al., 1992). A primary cause for concern among military personnel, who may be deployed on short notice, has been the risk of rebound scurvy due to sudden vitamin C withdrawal (Schrauzer and Rhead, 1973); however, clear evidence for this phenomenon is lacking. Likewise, the potential value of consumption from food sources rather than single-nutrient supplement intake requires greater study. However, the most prudent approach seems to be to increase fruit and vegetable consumption in the diet, thereby maximizing the potential benefits of antioxidant nutrients.

A factor that must be considered in recommending an increase in vitamin E intake is the level of PUFAs concomitantly being consumed in the diet. Increasing amounts of polyunsaturated fatty acids increase the vitamin E requirement because of the propensity of PUFAs to undergo lipid peroxidation. Approximately 0.4 mg of α-tocopherol equivalent for each gram of PUFA consumed has been suggested to be adequate in adult humans (Sokol, 1996).

Fatty Acids. Limited data suggest that moderate reductions in total fat calories (that is, 26 percent versus 30 percent) may have some beneficial effects in enhancing immune function. Increasing or decreasing the consumption of n-6 or n-3 PUFAs, or altering their intake ratios, may impact on immunological function. Although increased consumption of fish oils that supply eicosapentaenoic acid (EPA) and docosahexaenoic acid (DHA) may reduce the risk of heart disease and be beneficial in treating autoimmune diseases, their increased intake may reduce immune function, raise the dietary requirement for vitamin E, and affect blood clotting mechanisms (especially n-3 fatty acids).

Final Cautionary Notes. It is important to recognize that although modification of operational rations could potentially benefit the immune function of a large segment of the military population, a small but significant portion of the population could be harmed by such modifications because of genetic predisposition or other unknown factors. Also, it is possible that an elevated intake of a nutrient would result in a modification of immune function that is safe for a limited period but would diminish in safety or efficacy with prolonged use. Such a situation will necessitate a risk–benefit decision or the identification of a means by which to provide the supplemental nutrients in an additional ration component. Despite claims made by industry, some athletes, and sports coaches, most of the nutrients discussed in this report have failed thus far to demonstrate both safety and efficacy in modifying immune function, and further research is needed. Systematic studies should assess the extent to which subjects self-medicate with over-the-counter dietary food supplements, and such products should be evaluated carefully before their use is recommended.

5. Are there areas of investigation for the military nutrition research program that are likely to be fruitful in the sustainment of immune function in stressful conditions? Specifically, is there likely to be enough value added to justify adding to operational rations or including an additional component?

It is important to conduct research aimed at defining more specific nutrient–immune system interactions in order to elucidate the levels of key nutrients that are necessary to maintain proper immune function. Since these data also would be important for the general population, it is not necessary that this research be supported solely by the military; it could be conducted by other agencies. However, special studies of unique groups or circumstances (such as Ranger training) applying chiefly to the military might be warranted.

For some aspects of immune function, both beneficial and adverse effects related to nutrient intake may be encountered (some examples are vitamin A and iron). With this in mind, the CMNR suggests that the following areas are worthy of further investigation by the military nutrition research program:

• *Supplement use.* The military needs to gain a better understanding of supplement use by its personnel. Little information is available regarding the real benefits or potential toxic effects of nutritional supplements in supranormal amounts to warrant their further study for widespread use in the military at present. Indeed, some data indicate frank adverse effects of consuming one or more of these nutrients (such as copper and zinc) in pharmacologic amounts.

Although there seems to be relatively little risk associated with the use of vitamins C and E, and there may be relatively little risk associated with the use of β-carotene, major differences in potential benefits may exist between dietary exposure to such antioxidants and the use of supplements. Excessive supplementation with vitamin A, zinc, or selenium could prove toxic. The basis for this discrepancy and its impact on how such supplements are used should be addressed. In addition, the use of botanical and herbal supplements may be associated with risks that require further study.

• *Cytokines as an index of immune function.* As previously recommended by the CMNR (IOM, 1997), further research will be needed to determine if stress-related changes in cytokines can be detected reliably in spot urine samples collected during military field operations. Proinflammatory cytokines and their receptors and antagonists are all excreted in the urine. The magnitude of stress-related increases in the production of proinflammatory cytokines can be determined in whole-blood stimulation assays and possibly in 24-h urinary samples obtained during periods of stress, infectious illness, and/or trauma; however, the practicality and validity of urinary cytokine measures for field research studies must be determined.

Studies are necessary to determine if cytokine-related measurements have greater value, greater sensitivity, or greater stimulus-related specificity than the standard measurements of red blood cell sedimentation rates and CRP protein as indicators of systemic disease and/or as models of stress-induced release or suppression of proinflammatory cytokines.

• *Disease conditions and long-term host defense.* Ensuring prompt etiologic diagnosis of infectious illness and early therapy with effective antimicrobial agents will spare the loss of body nutrients by minimizing disease severity and duration. The severity and duration of fever are in proportion to measurable losses of nutrients from the body and/or their accelerated consumption. Accordingly, the control of high fevers (but not necessarily their total elimination) by specific drugs (ibuprofen, and to a lesser extent, aspirin) that prevent the conversion of arachidonic acid to fever-related eicosanoids (for example, the prostaglandins) will conserve body weight and nutrient stores. During protracted infections, nutritional supplements (multivitamin and/or multimineral pills, antioxidants, and amino acids such as glutamine and arginine) may provide valuable immunological support. The potential value of similar combinations of supplements, given as a possible prophylactic measure during periods of severe military stress, is currently unknown but warrants future study. Further, the consumption of high-quality diets should be encouraged early in convalescence to restore body nutrient pools and lost weight.

One important disease condition as yet unstudied is diarrhea. This condition should be examined to evaluate its effect on immune status indicators, both as a single variable and in combination with other important variables such as immunization, exercise, and reduced food intake. The major losses during diarrhea are those of water, sodium, potassium, and bicarbonate. None of these are known to have a direct effect on immune system functions; nonetheless, the resultant acidosis affects a variety of cell functions.

A key question involving the immune status of Special Forces troops is how acute nutrient deprivation during training may influence host defense on a long-term basis, and whether temporary nutritional and immune deficits incurred during training may produce long-term vulnerability (see recommendation in the CMNR's report of Ranger I studies [IOM, 1992]). Research also will be needed to determine if cytokine-induced losses of essential body nutrients are important concerns in military personnel exposed to other nonnutritional stresses.

• *Immune function in women.* Most studies to date have focused largely on male soldiers. Therefore, there is a paucity of information about the immune response of energy- and sleep-deprived female personnel who participate in training activities. Research is needed to evaluate the interrelationships among sleep, nutrition, physical activity, female sex hormone responses, menstrual cycle, and immune function in women in the military. An emerging area of interest is the evaluation of the effects of endogenous and exogenous (phyto- and xeno-) estrogens on immune function. Of particular importance are the deficiency of iron in many military women and the immunological consequences of iron deficiency.

CONCLUSIONS

The study of the interaction of nutrition and immune function is an exceptionally active area of research in both the military and the civilian (academic and commercial) sectors.

General Health Status

A considerable number of conditions encountered by the military act as immune stressors. These stressors include operationally induced undernutrition and dehydration; alterations in biological rhythms; atmospheric conditions such as temperature, humidity, and altitude; and environmental pollutants such as dust, smoke, and chemical fumes, as well as injuries and infectious agents themselves. As a result, studies of immune function in field situations contain many uncontrollable variables, and it is often difficult to attribute observed effects to one variable such as nutritional status.

The military's use of prophylactic immunization provides sufficient benefit beyond risk to warrant continued development. Recommendations concerning research on militarily relevant vaccines are contained in an earlier CMNR report (IOM, 1997). This is supported by a recent decision of the Secretary of Defense to begin systematic immunization of all U.S. military personnel against the biological warfare agent anthrax.

Pharmacologic agents such as aspirin, ibuprofen, and glucocorticoids modulate the effects of cytokines and can be used to minimize signs and symptoms of cytokine-induced acute-phase reactions and the nutrient losses that accompany them. Their use in military operations for the management of minor traumas and infections is well recognized and has been shown to sustain military performance during severe training exercises and operational missions.

Evidence to suggest that the administration of recombinant cytokines can modulate immune function in a desirable manner is limited at the present time to a small number of disease states. Their effectiveness has not been demonstrated in healthy subjects.

Field studies must be based on the results of prior experiments conducted in controlled laboratory and clinical settings. Experimental designs and methods must be validated by pilot tests prior to use. Because of the effects of circadian rhythms on immune function, samples must be collected at precisely defined times. In addition, because of the sensitivity and low levels of the molecules of interest, biological samples must be handled, transported, and stored according to recommendations for the materials in question, and appropriate controls must be included.

Nutritional Status

Total energy intake appears to play the greatest role in nutritional modulation of immune function. Since it has been demonstrated that prolonged energy deficits resulting in significant weight loss have an adverse effect on immune function, emphasis should be placed on the importance of adequate ration intake during military operations to minimize weight loss. Weight loss in the range of 10 percent in operations extending over 4 weeks raises the concern of reduced physical and cognitive performance and has potential health consequences for some individuals (IOM, 1995).

The nutritional status of soldiers should be optimized prior to deployment or engagement in any exercise or training course or even brief encounters with anything that would present a potential immune challenge (disease, toxic agent, or environmental stress). When consumed as recommended, operational rations provide adequate energy and macronutrients.

In addition to energy intake, nutrients that appear to play a role in immune function include protein, iron, zinc, copper, and selenium; the antioxidants β-carotene and vitamins C and E; vitamin A and the B-group vitamins, especially B$_6$, B$_{12}$, and folate; the amino acids glutamine and arginine; and the polyunsaturated fatty acids (PUFAs). It is difficult to consider the role of one nutrient in isolation. Evidence for a role for vitamin C in immunomodulation remains controversial, and the role of vitamin E has been demonstrated chiefly in the elderly. Available data also suggest that altered dietary intakes of essential polyunsaturated fatty acids (PUFAs), either the n-6 or the n-3 PUFAs, may influence immune functions. Iron deficiency impairs immune system competence and depresses the bactericidal functions of phagocytic cells. Excess iron as well as iron deficiency may also compromise immune status. Selenium deficiency is associated with increased susceptibility to particular infectious pathogens and may modify the virulence of a coxsackie virus that causes heart muscle damage. The latter observation may explain the apparent prevalence of Keshan disease, an endemic juvenile cardiomyopathy thought to be caused by a coxsackie virus, in areas of China experiencing periodic selenium deficiency. Glutamine has demonstrated potential for improving immune function in critical illness, and parenteral and enteral administration of glutamine has been observed to improve recovery following gastrointestinal surgery, but its usefulness in healthy populations has not been determined. Studies to evaluate the effects of supplemental glutamine on the immune function of soldiers have shown no demonstrable effects. The amounts of vitamins and trace elements (including zinc, copper, and selenium), contained in operational rations, meet all MRDAs (Military Recommended Dietary Allowances) if the diet is fully consumed. However, varying combinations of military stresses may increase the need for certain essential nutrients to values greater than the MRDA to maintain immunological competence.

Nutritional Supplements

The effects of providing supplements of vitamins A, C and E, as well as certain polyunsaturated fatty acids and amino acids, prior to, during, or following infections are virtually unknown in young, healthy adult men. Many questions remain regarding the efficacy of these nutrients in amounts that exceed Military Recommended Dietary Allowance (MRDA) levels. However, during protracted infections, nutritional supplements (multivitamin and/or multimineral pills, antioxidants, and amino acids such as glutamine and arginine) may provide valuable immunological support. Further, the consumption of high-quality diets should be encouraged early in convalescence to restore body nutrient pools and lost weight. *The most prudent approach seems to be one of increasing fruit and vegetable consumption in the diet, thus maximizing the potential benefits of antioxidant nutrients.*

Safety problems associated with excess consumption of supplements are much more likely for some nutrients than for others. Toxicity and the potential for nutrient–nutrient interactions must be considered individually. Excess intakes of vitamin A may be toxic, whereas vitamins C and E are relatively nontoxic and have been shown to enhance the immune response. Trace minerals are particularly problematic because requirements may be altered during periods of illness (increased), while at the same time, excessive intakes of some trace elements may be immunosuppressive.

Excess iron as well as iron deficiency may compromise immune status. The problem of compromised iron status in female personnel is a matter of concern because it may impact immune function, physical performance, and cognitive function. It is important to maintain adequate iron status in female soldiers and to do so without causing excess iron intake by males.

Glutamine has demonstrated potential for improving immune function in critical illness, but its usefulness in healthy populations is unknown. Parenteral and enteral administration of glutamine has been observed to improve recovery following gastrointestinal surgery. Thus far, the effect of glutamine has been observed only in supraphysiological amounts and only in patients undergoing bone marrow transplantation or major operations and those who sustain life-threatening sepsis. Studies to evaluate the effects of supplemental glutamine on the immune function of soldiers have shown no demonstrable effects. An effect of glutamine deficiency also has not been demonstrated.

Although none of the major body nutrients lost during severe diarrheal episodes (sodium, potassium, and bicarbonate) are known to influence immune function, rehydration strategies (and in some situations, supplementation with glutamine) may be of use in the treatment of diarrhea.

Finally, it must be emphasized that the results of studies performed in deficient animals or individuals are different from those done on adequately nourished ones and that, in many cases, an "overdose" of a nutrient, as well as a deficiency, leads to negative consequences.

RECOMMENDATIONS

Optimizing General Health Status

• **The CMNR recommends the use of medically appropriate and directed prophylactic medications and procedures to minimize the adverse effects of infectious agents. However, the CMNR sees no potential value at this time administering cytokines or anti-cytokines to healthy military personnel.**

It is generally assumed that the body's production of endogenous cytokines during stressful situations is beneficial to the host. However, if endogenous proinflammatory cytokines accumulate in large excesses or are given in large doses, they may have noxious or even dangerous consequences. The military should remain cognizant of the very active civilian-sector research concerning cytokines, their complex control mechanisms, and their functions, and should apply any pertinent new findings to the management of militarily relevant infectious diseases, trauma, or other stresses. The military should also keep apprised of advances (in the form of proven treatments) that emerge from this research.

• **In light of the importance of military immunization programs for achieving and maintaining immune status at optimal levels, the CMNR reiterates its previous recommendations (IOM, 1997) that vigorous research efforts be undertaken to create and evaluate militarily relevant oral vaccines.**

These should include optimization of administration schedules and elucidation of the influence of nutritional status on vaccine efficacy. Immunological responses to vaccines may be altered by the stresses of mobilization and/or overseas deployments. Antibody responses to vaccines are known to be depressed by protein-energy malnutrition. The potential problem of reduced responsiveness to military vaccines given during periods of mobilization and deployment stresses (in comparison to normal responses, as measured in control studies) also deserves future study.

• **It is recommended that soldiers maintain good physical fitness via a regular, moderate exercise program as a means of sustaining optimum immune function.** Since the intensity and duration of physical activity can affect immune function, training regimens that achieve high levels of physical fitness without adverse effects on immune status should be established.

• **Additionally, the CMNR recommends the use of methods to minimize psychological stresses, including training, conditioning, and structured briefing and debriefing.**

Optimizing Nutritional Status

• **In view of the compromised immune function noted in studies of Ranger trainees, the CMNR recommends that, where possible, individuals who have lost significant lean body mass should not be redeployed until this lean mass is regained.**

Although data showing an effect of weight loss on immune function may be limited, it is reasonable to suggest that the maintenance of body weight within 10 percent of ideal weight should increase the likelihood that adequate immune function will be maintained. Thus, the committee recommends that soldiers be advised to achieve an energy intake sufficient to maintain normal weight. The energy intakes required to maintain body weight will vary with the intensity and duration of physical activity; therefore, the best field guide for individual soldiers and commanders is to monitor body weight changes and to emphasize, through a "field-feeding doctrine," the importance of ration intake as the fuel for the soldier to maintain health and performance.

• **The CMNR recommends that nutritional anemia be treated prior to deployment and that individuals classified as anemic[1] and requiring iron supplements not be deployed.**

With the reduced personnel in today's Army and the potential for frequent deployment, it is important that soldiers be in good nutritional health at the time of deployment and that an effort be made to correct any compromise in status that may have resulted from previous deployment. Some scientists believe that iron supplements, if given during the course of bacterial or parasitic infections, may increase the severity of these illnesses. Because this topic is a controversial one, it requires further investigation. Nevertheless, it is recommended that if additional iron is required (for prophylactic purposes), it should be in the form of an optional ration supplement, and the iron content of operational rations themselves should not exceed MRDA levels.

• **As a means of reducing the number of stresses encountered by military personnel, the committee encourages the development and implementation of nutrition education programs targeted at high-risk military groups, such as Special Forces troops and female soldiers.**

The military should increase efforts to communicate information regarding healthy eating habits and supplement use to all personnel. Since dehydration and energy deficit have a great potential for compromising immune function, soldiers should also be educated regarding compliance with the "water doctrine."

Nutritional Supplement Use

Supplementation with certain nutrients may be of value for sustaining host defense mechanisms (including those conferred by the immune system) at normal levels during periods of extreme physiological and physical stress. Carefully controlled pilot and more extensive field studies will be necessary to investigate this possibility. It is unlikely, however, that nutritional supplements can produce a state of superimmunity in normal subjects or military personnel.

• **At this time, the CMNR cannot recommend general supplementation of military rations above the MRDAs for the purpose of enhancing immune function.**

---

[1] Iron deficiency anemia is defined as a serum ferritin concentration of less than 12 µg/ml in combination with a hemoglobin of less than 120 g/L.

There are no definitive studies that demonstrate positive benefits to young, healthy, active individuals of nutrient supplements at levels significantly in excess of those recommended by the MRDAs and commonly provided by foods. Encouraging ration intake to sustain nutrient levels as described in the MRDAs appears to be the best recommendation until further research clearly can define the likely benefits of specific nutrient supplementation under defined operational conditions. Soldiers should be cautioned regarding the indiscriminate use of individual supplements and the potential effects of inadequate nutrient intake, as well as the use of single or combined supplements, since their effects on immune status are not known.

• **The CMNR recommends that, when needed, the preferred method of providing supplemental nutrients is through a ration component.**

This would reduce both the potential for excessive intake by those individuals who do not need the nutrient and the potential misuse that exists when supplemental nutrients are provided in individual nutrient form. Because energy is one nutrient that has been identified as playing a role in immune function, provision of supplemental energy in the form of a food bar would allow soldiers to increase their nutrient intake as needed according to activity levels.

• **The CMNR recommends that the military gain a better understanding of supplement use as well as supplement abuse by personnel and make strong recommendations for the appropriate use or nonuse of nutritional supplements.**

The emphasis should be on education and wise choices. In the past, the CMNR has suggested the development of a "field-feeding doctrine" (IOM, 1995), with the guiding principle that the energy intakes of military personnel during training and combat operations should be adequate to meet their energy expenditures and to maintain body weight and lean body mass. This field-feeding doctrine would accompany the successful "water doctrine" that resulted from a recommendation in the report *Fluid Replacement in Heat Stress,* (IOM, 1991, 1993). The guiding principle of the water doctrine was to ensure that adequate fluid intake is maintained to avoid dehydration and subsequent decreased food intake. As more information is gained on supplement use and misuse and on the risks and benefits of supplements, the Army may want to consider formulating a "supplement doctrine" similar to the water and food doctrines to address these concerns and add a component to nutrition education programs. A better understanding of supplement use will provide information on the prevalence and frequency of use, its impact on an individual's nutritional status, and the likelihood of reckless or dangerous nutrition practices. Such information will help provide for the delivery of targeted and focused nutritional education messages. The committee is aware that some information on supplement use will be obtained by the Army Food and Nutrition Survey and suggests that additional information on supplement use can best be obtained by including appropriate questions in ongoing military health surveys, such as the Survey of Health-Related Behaviors Among Military Personnel.

Research Methodology

The CMNR strongly encourages the military to keep apprised of relevant civilian research and consider the application of selected findings and protocols to the military situation.

• **The CMNR recommends that research be conducted to determine the appropriate field measures for monitoring nutritionally induced immune responses, particularly for determining the presence of acute-phase reactions and changes in immune function of the type and degree that are likely to occur as a result of the nutritional insults suffered by soldiers in typical deployment situations.**

This will require basing field studies on appropriate clinical investigations, piloting experimental designs, and using a simple panel of standard tests that have been validated for the field. Particular attention must be paid to the timing of sample collection; the conditions under which samples are transported, stored, and handled; and the use of proper controls.

A rapid assessment of immune functions for use in the field includes clinical evaluations of local lesions, sites of inflammation, and signs and symptoms of generalized infectious illness. The C-reactive protein (CRP), erythrocyte sedimentation rate (ESR), and white cell counts are the most rapid and least expensive lab tests. Skin tests are highly valuable markers of cell-mediated immunity but require 48 hours before they can be read. Other tests can be valuable if time and facilities permit. On the other hand, preliminary clinical trials may employ additional kinds of sophisticated immunological studies, along with those listed for field investigations.

• **In addition, the CMNR recommends careful design of research protocols.**

Efforts should be directed towards ensuring the control of as many environmental, behavioral, and treatment variables as possible so that the effects attributed to a deficiency of a particular nutrient are not in fact the result of some other operational stress. The military nutrition research program should attempt to differentiate between nutrition-induced immune dysfunction and that caused by other forms of operational stress.

• **The CMNR strongly encourages the military to increase its awareness of and consider the military applications of the findings within the civilian research community regarding nutrition and immune function.** The advice of civilian and military immunologists should be sought to identify the testing methods that have proven to be most useful and field applicable for monitoring immune status and function.

RECOMMENDATIONS FOR FUTURE RESEARCH

Very little is yet known about the immunological effects of short-term food deprivation when accompanied by varying combinations of other military stresses. Future investigations into the changing immunological status of troops in the field must obviously be based upon available current knowledge about the immunological impact of individual stresses. However, because multiple stresses (including food deprivation) are to be expected, these will have to be studied using experimental designs and methods that have been validated by pilot studies prior to their use in large field studies.

• **The CMNR reiterates its previous recommendations (IOM, 1997) that *laboratory-based studies* be performed to determine if an interleukin-6 (IL-6)–creatinine ratio (or some comparable measure) can be measured in single "spot" urine samples as an index of the 24-h excretion of IL-6 and if 24-h IL-6 excretion is, in turn, a reliable indicator of acute stress response.**

Such determinations should be made before urinary IL-6 measurements are used in field studies, where 24-h urinary collections are virtually impossible to obtain.

• **The CMNR recommends the development and *field testing* of appropriate measurements of cytokines or their various markers in urine and blood that are reflective of ongoing acute-phase reactions and of changes in immune status in multistress environments.**

Developmental efforts should focus on one or two measurements that could be standardized with sufficient accuracy to serve as marker replacements for an entire (and complex) cytokine battery and would have some clinical correlate in immune function, such as skin test response and peak titer following vaccination. These may be useful in studies of the effects of nutritional status on immune function. Civilian research efforts in this area should be followed carefully, and collaborative relationships should be formed.

• **The CMNR recommends that if research is conducted on the ability of nutrients to influence immune status, priority at this time should be placed on the antioxidants β-carotene and vitamins C and E.**

The committee acknowledges that insufficient data are available to identify any specific nutrient or combination of nutrients as having adequately demonstrated the ability to enhance immune function under the military operational conditions investigated. This would include vitamins C and E, as well as the amino acids glutamine and arginine.

• **The influence of iron status on the risk of infection requires further investigation. This is also an area of interest to the civilian medical community.**

• **It is recommended that the military keep apprised of research being conducted in the civilian sector on immune function in physically active**

women and consider conducting studies on military women in situations of deployment to augment the findings of civilian studies.

At present, there are very few studies on the immune function of healthy women or women in high stress situations.

The Committee on Military Nutrition Research is pleased to participate with the Military Nutrition Division, U.S. Army Research Institute of Environmental Medicine, and the U.S. Army Medical Research and Materiel Command in progress relating to the nutrition, performance, and health of U.S. military personnel.

REFERENCES

DeRijk, R.H., J. Petrides, P. Deuster, P.W. Gold, and E.M. Sternberg. 1996. Changes in corticosteroid sensitivity of peripheral blood lymphocytes after strenuous exercise in humans. J. Clin. Endocrinol. Metab. 81(1):228–235.

DeRijk, R., D. Michelson, B. Karp, J. Petrides, E. Galliven, P. Deuster, G. Paciotti, P.W. Gold, and E.M. Sternberg. 1997. Exercise and circadian rhythm-induced variations in plasma cortisol differentially regulate interleukin-1β (IL-1β), Il-6, and tumor necrosis factor-α (TNFα) production in humans: High sensitivity of TNFα and resistance of IL-6. J. Clin. Endocrinol. Metab. 82(7):2182–2191.

IOM (Institute of Medicine). 1991. Fluid Replacement and Heat Stress, 3d printing., B.M. Marriott, ed. A report of the Committee on Military Nutrition Research, Food and Nutrition Board. Washington, D.C.: National Academy Press.

IOM. 1992. A Nutritional Assessment of U.S. Army Ranger Training Class 11/91. A brief report of the Committee on Military Nutrition Research, Food and Nutrition Board. March 23, 1992. Washington, D.C.

IOM. 1993. Nutritional Needs in Hot Environments, Applications for Military Personnel in Field Operations, B.M. Marriott, ed. A report of the Committee on Military Nutrition Research, Food and Nutrition Board, Washington, D.C.: National Academy Press.

IOM. 1995. Not Eating Enough, Overcoming Underconsumption of Military Operational Rations, B.M. Marriott, ed. A report of the Committee on Military Nutrition Research, Food and Nutrition Board. Washington, D.C.: National Academy Press.

IOM. 1997. Emerging Technologies for Nutrition Research, Potential for Assessing Military Performance Capability, S.J. Carson-Newberry and R.B. Costello, eds. A report of the Committee on Military Nutrition Research, Food and Nutrition Board. Washington, D.C.: National Academy Press.

Mackowiak, P.A., J.G. Bartlett, E.C. Borden, S.E. Goldblum, J.D. Hasday, R.S. Munford, S.A. Nasraway, P.D. Stolley, and T.E. Woodward. 1997. Concepts of fever: Recent advances and lingering dogma. Clin. Infect. Dis. 25:119–138.

Newhouse, I.J., and D.B. Clement. 1988. Iron status in athletes. An update. Sports Med. 5:337–352.

Schrauzer, G.N., and W.J. Rhead. 1973. Ascorbic acid abuse: effects on long term ingestion of excessive amounts on blood levels and urinary excretion. Int. J. Vitam. Nutr. Res. 43(2):201–211.

Sokol, R.J. 1996. Vitamin E. Pp. 130–136 in Present Knowledge in Nutrition, 7th ed., E. Khard, E. Ziegler, and L.J. Filer, eds. Washington, D.C.: ILSI Press.

Straight, J.M., H.M. Kipen, R.F. Vogt, and R.W. Amler. 1994. Immune Function Test Batteries for Use in Environmental Health Studies. U.S. Department of Health and Human Services, Public Health Service. Publication Number: PB94-204328.

Westphal K.A., A.E. Pusateri, and T.R. Kramer. 1994. Prevalence of negative iron nutriture and relationship with folate nutriture, immunocompetence, and fitness level in U.S. Army servicewomen. USARIEM Approved Protocol OPD94002-AP024-H016. Defense Women's Health Research Program 1994, Log No. W4168016. Natick, Mass.: U.S. Army Research Institute of Environmental Medicine.

Westphal, K.A., L.J. Marchitelli, K.E. Friedl, and M.A. Sharp. 1995. Relationship between iron status and physical performance in female soldiers during U.S. Army basic combat training. Fed. Am. Soc. Exp. Biol. J. 9(3):A361[abstract].

WHO (World Health Organization). 1996. Trace Elements in Human Nutrition and Health. Geneva: WHO.

Appendix M

Conclusions and Recommendations from the Workshop Report The Role of Protein and Amino Acids in Sustaining and Enhancing Performance

Submitted June 1999

Committee Responses to Questions, Conclusions, and Recommendations

As presented in the Executive Summary of this report, The Committee on Military Nutrition Research (CMNR) in collaboration with its Subcommittee on Body Composition, Nutrition, and Health was requested to update findings in earlier CMNR reports (IOM, 1992, 1994, 1995) with respect to the role of protein and amino acids in maintaining and enhancing the physical and cognitive performance of soldiers. The committee's conclusions and recommendations are provided below as part of the response to the three specific questions posed by the military.

1. Do protein requirements increase with military operational stressors, including high workload with or without energy deficit? Are there gender differences in protein requirements in endurance exercise?

At the present time, controversy exists regarding the validity of recent estimations of protein and amino acid requirements (particularly the latter) for adults, a controversy that is based on methodological questions.

In addition, the evidence that high levels of physical activity increase protein requirements for individuals whose energy intake matches their output is equivocal. There is clear evidence that moderate physical activity increases the efficiency of protein utilization. However, strenuous endurance-type exercise has been shown to increase protein requirements above the recommended dietary allowance (RDA), but not the Military Recommended Dietary

Allowance (MRDA). In contrast, resistance exercise does not appear to increase the requirement for maintenance of lean mass, although the protein intake that would be required for active individuals to increase tissue mass (1.2–1.5 g/kg BW/d) may be higher than that for sedentary individuals. There is also strong evidence that the efficiency of protein utilization is decreased (and the requirements increased) by a state of negative energy balance.

However, much of the research on the effects of physical activity on protein requirements and the effects of altered protein intakes on performance is difficult to interpret because of the time required for the body to adapt to changes in protein intake. One implication of this adaptation that is of concern for service personnel is that continuous excessive intake of protein may cause increased protein catabolism, resulting in greater risk when protein intake is reduced.

Systemic infection and serious injuries clearly increase protein requirements. However, data suggest that in patients recovering from burns or any major trauma, an increase in dietary protein intake does not permit the recovery of muscle mass to begin immediately, due to the acute-phase response, which is accompanied by changes in hormonal status. Longer term studies are therefore needed during recovery periods. Research on the effects of treatment with anabolic hormones, which stimulate protein synthesis or decrease protein breakdown, is ongoing.

Results of studies of protein requirements in hot, cold, and high-altitude environments suggest that these conditions do not increase protein requirements beyond currently recommended levels. In addition, because increases in protein intake also increase fluid requirements and sources of fluid for drinking are often limited during operations in extreme environments, previous reports of the Committee on Military Nutrition Research (CMNR) have cautioned against excessive protein intake under such circumstances.

The effects of combined stressors and other factors such as emotional stress on protein requirements have not been documented.

As emphasized in earlier IOM reports (IOM, 1992, 1995), the importance of adequate energy intake (sufficient to match output and avoid weight loss) and protein intake should be emphasized to soldiers as the primary means of maintaining lean tissue mass. Research is needed to resolve the controversy regarding the adult requirement for indispensable amino acids and to quantitate more precisely the effect of energy deficit on protein and indispensable amino acid requirements.

Military researchers and physicians should pay careful attention to civilian research on the effects of treatment with anabolic hor-

mones on recovery from burns and other injuries. Where appropriate, military-specific models should be developed.

2. What is the optimal protein content (and protein-to-energy ratio) for standard operational rations, and specifically, is the Military Recommended Dietary Allowance for operational rations (100 g/d for men and 80 g/d for women) appropriate? Is the protein MRDA for women appropriate during pregnancy and lactation?

Without more data on the functional implications of varying protein intakes, it is not possible to define with accuracy the optimal protein content of standard operational rations. However, based on currently available data, the use of the MRDA for operational rations is appropriate and provides a generous level of protein intake. The MRDA covers the protein requirements of pregnant and lactating women.

Current MRDAs for protein should be maintained. Provided that energy intake is adequate, no increase in MRDAs is necessary for pregnant or lactating women.

3. Is there evidence that supplementation with specific amino acids (AAs) or modification of dietary protein quality would optimize military performance, either cognitive or physical, during high workload, psychological stress, or energy deficit. What are the risks of amino acid supplements and high-protein diets?

At the present time, considerable debate surrounds the adult requirement for indispensable amino acids and thus high-quality proteins. Research fails to support the use of protein supplements to facilitate muscle building or improve physical performance under conditions of adequate energy and protein intake. In addition, research supporting the use of tyrosine supplements to enhance cognitive performance under field conditions is inconclusive. Supplemental glutamine and arginine have yet to show conclusively beneficial effects on immune function. The MRDA, if consumed, provides adequate protein and energy to sustain immune function under normal field conditions. Furthermore, with the exception of tryptophan, commercial preparations of which have been documented to cause specific toxic effects, there is a lack of safety data on the consumption of high levels of individual amino acids.

Some plant proteins such as those from soy and other legumes have an adequate balance of essential amino acids to meet the protein needs of military personnel. These plant foods may have the advantage of decreasing the risk of cardiovascular disease due to their content of soluble carbohydrates, their lower sodium and lower fat contents, and the presence of other as yet unidentified substances.

Current intakes of protein among military populations are high and show no apparent harmful effects, provided fluid intake is adequate. There is little evidence of increased health risks from a high intake of dietary protein; however, an amino acid imbalance may be created with the use of single amino acid or protein supplements. Although no data are available from groups similar in age and fitness characteristics to military personnel, a review of the information available shows that high protein intake is not associated with direct effects on renal dysfunction, although high-protein diets may indirectly stimulate renal stone formation and result in an increased renal workload because of the need to concentrate urine. High protein intake has been shown to increase urinary calcium loss, but there is no definitive evidence that the level of protein intake observed in Army women in field conditions represents a risk factor for osteoporosis.

> **Given adequate nutritional intake, soldiers should not use protein supplements for muscle building. Military researchers and physicians should pay careful attention to civilian research on the use of anabolic hormones to increase muscle or lean tissue mass.**

> **Protein supplied in operational rations should be of high quality and digestibility. Energy intakes should be adequate, and sources of energy should be consumed within 2 hours of an intense bout of endurance exercise, to replace depleted muscle glycogen.**

> **Soy food products are a healthful substitute for animal-based products; however individual products should be tested for their acceptability to soldiers.**

> **Single amino acid supplements should not be used to modify cognitive performance, due to potential toxicity and insufficient evidence of efficacy.**

> **The military should test the ability of supplemental glutamine and arginine to enhance the immune response and decrease rates of infection under field conditions and in seriously injured hospitalized patients.**

> **Given the high protein content of operational rations, adequate fluid intake should be emphasized, as recommended by the "Fluid Doctrine" (IOM, 1994).**

REFERENCES

IOM (Institute of Medicine). 1992. A Nutritional Assessment of U.S. Army Ranger Training Class 11/91. March 23. Washington, D.C.

IOM. 1994. Food Components to Enhance Performance, An Evaluation of Potential Peformance-Enhancing Food Components for Operational Rations, B.M. Marriott, ed. Washington, D.C.: National Academy Press.

IOM. 1995. Not Eating Enough, Overcoming Underconsumption of Military Operational Rations, B.M. Marriott, ed. Washington, D.C.: National Academy Press.